Instant Teaching Tools

for

Health Care Educators

Instant Teaching Tools

for

Health Care Educators

Michele L. Deck, MEd, BSN, RN, ACCE-R

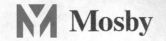 Mosby

An Affiliate of Elsevier Science

St. Louis   London   Philadelphia   Sydney   Toronto

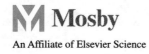
Mosby

An Affiliate of Elsevier Science

Mosby, Inc.
11830 Westline Industrial Drive
St. Louis, Missouri 63146

Library of Congress Cataloging-in-Publication Data
Deck, Michele.
     Instant teaching tools for health care educators / Michele Deck.
        p.   cm.
     Includes bibliographical references (p.   ).
     ISBN 0-8151-2379-5 (pbk.)
     1. Health education.   I. Title
   RA440.5.D43   1995
   610'.71—dc20

                                  94-48054

02 / 9 8 7

Michele Deck
MEd, BSN, RN, ACCE-R

Michele has been training adults for over thirteen years. She received her Bachelor of Science degree in nursing from Louisiana State University Medical Center in New Orleans and a master's degree in adult education from the University of Southern Mississippi. Michele began her fourteen-year nursing career as a nurse's aide on a medical surgical unit, then progressed to hospital obstetric nursing. She is an ASPO Certified Childbirth Educator and has maintained a thriving independent Lamaze practice for over ten years. Michele has been in staff development at all levels of nursing service personnel for the last six years. She has taught topics from orientation to mandatory training for JCAHO to CPR and advanced life support. She won the prestigious "Excellence in Nursing" award at her hospital two years in a row. She was also selected as a "Great 100 Nurse in Louisiana" in 1989 and was elected to Sigma Theta Tau National Nursing Honor Society in 1990. Michele has found time to be a Senior Training Consultant for Creative Training Techniques International, Inc. since 1989.

Michele is known for her innovative teaching methods in the field of health care education. In February of 1989, the *Journal of Pediatric Nursing* published her article "The Games We Play." In May of 1990, Creative Training Techniques International, Inc. published her manual *Getting Adults Motivated, Enthusiastic and Satisfied*, based on her experience using television game shows as a method of instruction for technical information. She has been cited with her coauthor Jeanne R. Silva in eight separate issues of *Creative Training Techniques Newsletter*, an internationally circulated newsletter by Lakewood Publications. Her two latest collaborations are called *Presenter's Survival Kit: It's a Jungle Out There* and *Instant Teaching Tools For Health Care Educators*. Michele is the co-owner of a nursing education consulting firm in Metairie, Louisiana, called G.A.M.E.S. (Gimics and Mania Educate Staff). Her latest venture is a creative product company called Tool Thyme for Trainers that features items to make repetitive sessions fun for all.

In 1992 Michele presented at the American Society for Training and Development's (ASTD) national conference. She conducted a preconference session at the 1991 American Society for Healthcare Education and Training's (ASHET) national conference where she was one of the highest rated speakers. Her presentations at Resource Applications Staff Development conferences in February 1992, 1993, and 1994 had standing room only. Michele has been on the national faculty of Lakewood Publication's Total Trainer conference for the last four years. In 1994 she presented a preconference for the American Association of Critical Care Nurses and a Congress session at the National Association of Operating Room Nurses.

Contributors

Rosalie Barker, BSN, RNC
Clinical Educator
Ochsner Foundation Hospital
New Orleans, LA

Barbara Bonheur, MS, RN
Coordinator of the
Community Health Programs
International Medical
Education Curriculum
Operation Smile International
Norfolk, VA

**Linda Brazen, MSN, RN,
C, CNOR**
Continuing Education Coordinator
Center for Perioperative Education
Association of
Operating Room Nurses, Inc.
Denver, CO

Lana Brumfield, BSN, RN
Staff Nurse
Ochsner Foundation Hospital
New Orleans, LA

Mary Arnone Cahoon, BS, RN
Staff Development and
Training Coordinator
Community Health and
Counseling (Health Services)
Bangor, ME

**Jann Christensen, MPA,
BSN, RN**
Director of Education
Midwestern Regional
Medical Center
Zion, IL

Joanne Clovis, BSN, RN
Educator
St. Alphonse Regional
Medical Center
Boise, ID

Martha Dardenne, BSN, RN
Clinical Educator
Ochsner Foundation Hospital
New Orleans, LA

Joanne Ekstedt, BSN, RN, ICCE
Educational Specialist
Lee Memorial Hospital
Cape Coral, FL

**Janet Fitts, BSN, RN, CEN,
EMT-P**
Firefighter/Paramedic/
Registered Nurse
Eureka Fire Protection District
Eureka, MO

Linnea Frey, MS, RN
Director of Education and Exhibits
Health Adventure Center
Columbia, MO

Marty Grove, BS, RN
Instructor, Educational Services
Mercy Hospital Anderson
Cincinnati, OH

Sherry Haizlip, BSN, RN, C
Clinical Education Coordinator
Medical Center of Central Georgia
Macon, GA

Nancy Hennen, BSN, RNC
Clinical Educator
Ochsner Foundation Hospital
New Orleans, LA

**Gretchen Hrachovec, MA,
BSN, RNC**
Education Specialist
Hillcrest Medical Center
Tulsa, OK

continued

Contributors *continued*

Tina Johnson, BS
Professional Recruiting Specialist
Carle Clinic
Urbana, IL

Mary LaBiche, MEd, RRT
Program Director, Program in
Respiratory Care
Ochsner School of Allied
Health Sciences
New Orleans, LA

**Bonnie Maestri, MN,
RNC, ACCE**
Instructor
Loyola City College
Nursing Program
New Orleans, LA

**Amanda Martin, MEd, BSN,
RN, CNOR**
Ochsner Foundation Hospital
Clinical Educator
New Orleans, LA
Consultant—ATM Consultants
Harahan, LA

Phyllis J. Miller, MS, RN, FHCE
Director, Center for
Nursing Education
Greater Southeast
Community Hospital
Washington, DC

Cheri Penas, MS, RN, CCRN
Educator
MeritCare Medical Center
Education Services
Fargo, ND

**Regina Lawless Phelps,
MN, RN**
Director of Nursing Education
and Research
Ochsner Foundation Hospital
New Orleans, LA

Lanelle Picarella, MEd, RN
Clinical Educator
Ochsner Foundation Hospital
New Orleans, LA

Joan Prokop-Roberts, MN, RN
Staff Development Instructor
Natividad Medical Center
Salinas, CA

Theresa Rimer, BSN, RN, CPN
Phoenix, AZ

**Raeleen Roberts, MSN, RN,
CCRN**
Education Coordinator
North Chicago VA Medical Center
North Chicago, IL

Susan B. Roders, BSN, RN
Nurse Educator
Sacred Heart Health System
Eugene, OR

Linda Rodriguez
Computer Trainer
Ochsner Foundation Hospital
New Orleans, LA

**Julie Sandstrom, MS, RN,
CCRN**
Registered Nurse
MeritCare Medical Center
Education Services
Fargo, ND

Kathy Sciborski, MLT, (ASCP)
Lab Coordinator
Lutheran Hospital LaCrosse
LaCrosse, WI

**Miriam Sheridan, EdD,
MN, RN**
Associate Chief Nurse for
Education and Research
Biloxi VA Medical Center
Biloxi, MS

continued

Contributors *continued*

Jeanne Silva, BSN, RN, CCRN
Consultant
Gimics and Mania Educate Staff
Metairie, LA

**Susan Thornton, MEd,
RN, CEN**
Education Coordinator
Forsyth Memorial Hospital
Winston-Salem, NC

**Kim Major Walker, MSN,
RN, CCRN**
Apex, NC

Suzi Weigel, MA
Program Director, Fitness
St. Vincent's Wellness Services
Carmel, IN

Nancy Wilson, MSN, RN
Director of Education
Clermont Mercy Hospital
Batavia, OH

Nancy Yentzen, MS, RNC
Nurse Educator
Memorial Hospital at Gulfport
Gulfport, MS

Preface

Let me invite you to take an educational journey into the creative side of your mind. This is the part of your brain that enjoys a challenge, likes to have fun, and is proud when you make a difference in someone's life. How do we as health care educators make a difference in the lives of our students? We do it every day, so sometimes we take it for granted. Most often it affects the lives and careers of the health care personnel we teach. Some might approach teaching with dread; others with, "Oh, no, not again!" But some of us have discovered a magical secret.

It may be the 1,346th time we have taught a topic, but it is the special first time some of our participants learn it. The session becomes a once-in-a-lifetime event from their viewpoint. Wow! What an opportunity for us to give them our best! I know what you're thinking. What about those times when they have seen and heard it before? They are prisoners of curriculum or mandatory sessions. What then?

The repetitive sessions push us, as educators, to extend our teaching abilities. We are confident in knowing the content, so we can try some new ways to teach it. This is what keeps us fresh and helps us to grow. Always trying one new method or idea can make a session terrific! It's also our opportunity to continually improve what we do and to develop our talents.

Here is the real secret. When we assist others in furthering their knowledge and improving their attitudes and skills, we affect their lives. We touch people at an important and personal level by increasing their ability to do their jobs effectively. What bigger effect is there in the universe than touching someone else's life? I can't think of anything! So, I now invite you to embark on a fun, different, and meaningful creative journey. Along the way you will learn more about yourself and the way you teach.

There are some ready-to-use instant ideas in this book. Some require just a small amount of personalization to your organization or learners. Others may spark a completely new idea for you to develop independently. There is a page at the end of the book on which you may suggest methods you have used successfully for volume two of *Instant Teaching Tools for Health Care Educators*.

A goal of mine in writing this book was to make it as easy to use as possible. One way to do that was to eliminate the titles on each of the tool pages. Instead of the words, time frame, how-tos, and so forth, there are symbols containing information. Let this book be your first and most important step in beginning your own creative journey. *Bon Voyage!*

—*Michele Deck*

▶▶

Acknowledgments

Thank you a million times over to the special people who made this book a reality. Thank you to Jackie Katz, a visionary in the field of health care education. Jackie's creativity and determination made this book possible. I am truly fortunate to have met Jackie and Jay Katz, and I enjoy the opportunities they continue to offer me. Thank you to Barb Watts for her patience and attention to detail in handling the manuscript.

Thank you to all of those highly creative and totally unselfish people who contributed ideas for this book. The generosity of Regina Phelps deserves special recognition. She is a nursing leader who encouraged me and many others to develop our creativity, even coming to our defense in the initial growing pains. More than half the ideas in this book were developed in her Nursing Education and Research Department at Ochsner Foundation Hospital, and she graciously shares them, as well as her personal ideas, here. Regina, thanks for the many gifts you have given to me!

Thank you to Jeanne Silva, my education mentor, and to Nancy Hennen, who allowed me to mentor her in some small way. Each taught me much about the joy and fun of learning with challenging content, learners, and environment. Thank you to Amanda Martin, the brightest and most determined person I know. Thank you, Pamela Brown-Stewart! You have opened many doors to me, including those to your super ideas and friendship.

Thank you to the health care educators who shared their ideas with Mosby's contest and my request. I am inspired by the innovation in our field and by the willingness of these extraordinary people who are sharing it here. Thank you for trusting me with your ideas, even though some of us have met only by phone or letter. Please pardon the changes and personalizations to your ideas, which were made to simplify the use of this book. Thank you, Miriam, Mary, Raeleen, Gretchen, Jann, Susan, Lynn, Bonnie, Theresa, Julie, Cheri, Barbara, Nancy, Joanne, Janet, Joan, Kim, Kathy, Linda, Tina, Suzi, Sherry, Rosie, Martha, Lanelle, Marty, Phyllis, and Lana. Thank you, one and all!

Thank you to Lori Backer who has taught me to be a million times more visual and creative. I'd like to be as talented as you when I grow up. Thank you for the visual layout ideas. You are terrific! Thank you to Bob Pike for the creative opportunities he offered me. He is the definitive example of living one's dream. I thank you for the personal and professional examples.

Last, but not least, thank you to my loving and wonderful husband Brian and our daughters Melissa, Melanie, and Brittany. A more supportive family does not exist in the universe. I love you and appreciate your always loving and understanding resilience to whatever comes in our life. This book is dedicated to you.

—*Michele Deck*

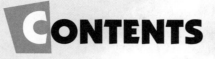

CONTENTS

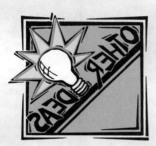

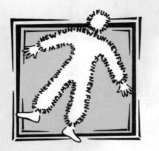
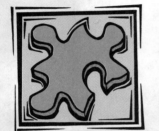
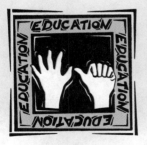
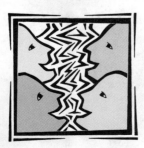

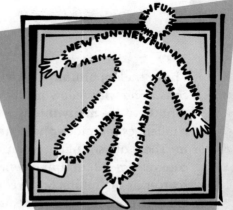

PART 1

CHALLENGES WE SHARE

CHALLENGES WE SHARE

Limited Resources

I have the opportunity to travel throughout the United States meeting and consulting with fellow health care educators. I was at first surprised to find that there are many things we have in common. We seem to face the same challenges, no matter how large or small our facility or which state we live in. There are shrinking resources of time, money, and people. With health care reform still an unknown, many fear that resources will become even scarcer in the future. Some educators complain that they would like to use creative approaches to teaching content but that their preparation time is limited. They are too busy solving crises to devote time to creative program design and prop making. Many institutions have one-person departments or faculty.

It is truly a challenge to have ongoing content sessions, while working in a staff job as well. Some who are not familiar with the job of educator are unaware of the 80/20 rule of course preparation: 80 percent of time is spent in preparation, only 20 percent of the time is in the classroom, that is, the actual course length. If an educational session is eight hours in length (one day), it takes at least four days of preparation time, or thirty-two hours, for development and planning. This is a conservative estimate, considering the intensity and importance of our health care content.

Saving Time

This is the very reason these instant tools were conceived. Many of the tools have READY-TO-USE pages that are designed to be copied for *instant* usability. (These pages are indicated by a boxed check-mark located in the upper outer corner.) Some ideas may take up to fifteen to thirty minutes to customize to best fit a particular health care topic or group.

Most of these educational activities are brief, requiring from just five minutes to one hour of classroom time. As these high involvement lessons may be more memorable, we may actually save time in the long run. We will be using highly effective teaching methods that build retention, so that we spend less time in repeating our lessons verbally.

Tradition

Tradition may dictate that we primarily use lecture to teach. After all, isn't that what we are familiar with? Isn't lecture the method our teachers used to teach us? Isn't this the way it has always been? Educational research has shown that for the 1990s learner, lecture is an ineffective way to share information. David G. Jensen of the UCLA School of Medicine confirms in "The Science of Effective Presentations" that traditional lecture is not the most effective method of teaching.* We live in a highly visual age in which our learners are the television and video generation. They are accustomed to a visual variety, and just talking to this group does not hold their attention. Our learners have been unconsciously conditioned to seek variety, involvement, and change at short intervals. Does lecture invite high involvement and change often? It does not. I believe many educators themselves have not experienced a variety of learning methods and therefore fall back on the familiar and comfortable lecture. But who has not lectured and been frustrated seeing bored faces and inattentive eyes? Some of us are looking for new, more effective ways to teach than this.

Results Based

Why should we use these creative tools? They are based on adult education theory and practice. Using them works. These are results-based tools that reinforce learning. Telling information does not ensure that it has been learned. Lecture is instructor-focused, not learner-focused.

When we have limited resources, is there time to use ineffective methods? We must be as effective as possible as quickly as possible. We must teach with outcomes in mind: "The learner will be able to . . . ." versus "Here is some important information about . . . ." Part of being results-based includes planning follow-up, reinforcing, and measuring. Repetition and reinforcement equal retention for learners. Some of the tools used here are fun, produce no more than low anxiety, and have sneaky review formats.

Professionalism

Some might argue that these tools are too much fun to be "professional." What is professionalism in learning? Is it using the most effective tools and methods available, always striving to become a better educator, and being willing to take a learning risk? If so, then these tools are completely professional, because they met these criteria. Some educators say, "What if someone laughs at me?" Relax and enjoy the process with them. Don't worry. Act as if this is fun for you also. Sometimes you might want to laugh at yourself if it helps someone to learn! We must be mindful of our ultimate goal: that our learners learn. There are many highly paid business and industry professionals who use the same kinds of tools for the same reason. We in health care can set our own trends and be in step with new and innovative ideas as they are developed.

---

*From Jensen DG: The science of effective presentations, Los Angeles, 1993, UCLA School of Medicine (graduate thesis).

Familiar Formats

Most of these instant tools use familiar formats for activities in order to cut down on the explanation time. There are ready-to-use pages with explanations that are available to copy and immediately use. The less time spent explaining means more time learning. Some formats look like games we have played. Some are modified television-type game shows; others are old favorites such as cards, crossword puzzles, bingo, and so forth. These are quick and fun ways to reinforce content without having the learner become bored and uninvolved in the lesson. The learner relaxes and enjoys the activity, breaking through the anxiety barrier and learning without focusing on how much he or she is absorbing.

Building Memory

The physiology of memory is important in planning learning experiences. The brain operates in three domains during learning. The first domain controls the autonomic functions and is located in the brain stem. It affects our basic functions. The midbrain acts as the air traffic controller and decides what information moves into long-term memory. The upper brain involves the cerebral cortex where complex and conscious thought occurs.

If learners are anxious, the flight-or-fright reaction occurs. This anxiety does not allow the higher brain functions to readily operate but interferes by creating a phenomenon called *downshifting*. This interrupts all conscious thoughts. Have you ever seen learners so nervous that facts pass over their heads? Emotions play a role in this memory process. If we have positive feelings about an experience, we tend to remember it. For example, can you remember a great day in your life? We also remember those negative occurrences in our life. Can you think of a bad day you had in the recent past? Now, can you remember the price per pound of apples last March? Most people will not remember that fact for two reasons. It is neither a positive nor a negative feeling for them. It is routine or "ho-hum." If our learners' experiences are positive and happy, they will remember them. If they hate the session, they will remember enough of it to complain in detail to those who will listen.

So, how can we increase the possibility that the midbrain will move the information to long-term memory? Give our learners a positive and fun experience! If they have a negative experience, they will remember it, but we won't have jobs for long! If it is the same old lecture format, it will pass right through the "air traffic controller" midbrain without notice, not into memory.

Serious Content

Some people raise the issue that it's impossible to make serious content fun. The more serious the content, the more crucial it is to lower anxiety while raising retention. We therefore can choose to use a high involvement and enjoyable activity to get our message across. Select the most important, crucial-to-know information and competencies, and use the high retention tools in this book to teach them. This will help commit the information to the recall area of memory. After all, if the learners can't recall crucial content, how will they use it? To increase your comfort level, at first choose a tool that is low risk for your learners and for you. Select one idea that looks as if it would appeal to your learners. Use it several times before incorporating another idea. Must you completely revamp all your lessons overnight? No, but choosing to use one new idea each time you teach the same content is a good plan.

Repetition

Another challenge we share is the repetitive nature of our content. It is sometimes difficult to be happy and energetic about content we have taught many times. If we are not excited about our content, our learners never will be! These tools can be interesting and invigorating for the educator. Fun re-energizes you and prevents burnout. It can revitalize your approach to familiar content. In refreshing yourself, you may discover a more effective way to teach a block of content. Mixing and matching methods and content prevents educators from having the same day over and over again each time they conduct a session. Where can we obtain different ideas for methods? We can trade ideas with colleagues, read this book and others like it, or sometimes invent a great idea ourselves. All it takes is a small amount of creativity and an adventurous spirit. On the following pages are many ideas you can use to begin revitalizing your teaching.

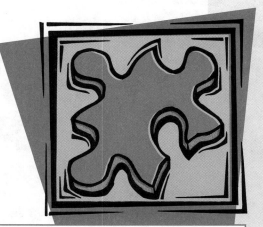

PART 2

INSTANT TOOLS FOR MANDATORIES

20 minutes

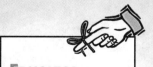

TOOL BOX

4 signs (Work
Environment, Body
Mechanics, Fall
Prevention, and
Needle Stick
Prevention Safety
Measures), pens or
pencils, Safety
Measures Match
fill-in-the-blank
sheets, answer key,
safety certificates

SAFETY MEASURES MATCH

Preparation

1. Copy the ready-to-use sheet listing the four safety measures, and cut the sheet into four sections. Copy each section on a differently colored sheet of paper.

2. Copy as many Safety Measures Match fill-in-the-blank sheets as there are participants. Copies should be on the same colored paper you used for the signs, divided as equally as possible among the four colors.

3. Make sure each participant has a pen or pencil.

4. Have the answer key available for checking answers.

5. Copy a safety certificate for each attendee. (Safety certificate is ready to use on page 13.)

6. Place one category sign in each corner of the room.

Implementation

1. Explain that you will focus on four safety categories (work environment, body mechanics, fall prevention, and needle stick prevention).

2. Distribute the fill-in-the-blank sheets to each participant.

3. Read aloud this explanation statement: "This is an activity that will help us examine safety issues we see every day in patient care activities. Your job is to fill in the blanks on the page with the choices listed in the right column. Use each word only once."

4. Ask the participants to go to the corner with the colored sign that matches the color of their fill-in-the-blank sheet.

5. Have each group pick a safety captain.

continued

EDUCATOR SECRETS:

Check the five
answers the groups
have selected before
they report to the
entire room.

By: Rosalie Barker, BSN, RNC
Nancy Hennen, BSN, RNC

SAFETY MEASURES MATCH *continued*

6. The group discusses the answers and makes sure each member's blanks are filled in.

7. The safety captains help their group identify which five safety measures of the twenty are related to their group's safety category (this appears on their sign).

8. The instructor circulates among the groups to make sure the five safety measures selected are correct and to answer questions and clarify categories.

9. The safety captains then read their five selections to the entire group.

10. The instructor may elaborate on any points he or she feels are pertinent.

11. Everyone receives a safety certificate at the end.

Safety Measures Match

Directions: Cut out boxes below and copy each onto colored paper.

Work Environment Safety Measures

Body Mechanics Safety Measures

Fall Prevention Safety Measures

Needle Stick Prevention Safety Measures

SAFETY MEASURES MATCH

Directions: Match each of the **key terms** to the appropriate safety measure.

Safety Measures

1. Wipe up _____ immediately and call house-keeping if necessary.

2. _____ instead of bending to pick up heavy objects from the floor.

3. Empty sharps containers when _____.

4. Return the bed to the _____ after patient care.

5. Everyone is responsible for maintaining a safe _____.

6. Place the full sharps container in the _____.

7. _____ when transferring patients.

8. Remove _____ and equipment from patient rooms.

9. _____ at risk for falling with activities.

10. Avoid _____ sharps containers.

11. Identify _____ for falls.

12. Rolling equipment needs to be _____ of the hall.

13. Never _____ needles.

14. Place the _____ within the patient's reach.

15. Label _____ and notify appropriate department.

16. When carrying objects hold them _____.

17. Raise _____ on beds when necessary.

18. Stand with your feet apart to maintain a proper _____.

19. Always _____ sharps container's lid upon disposal.

20. _____ instead of lifting whenever possible.

Key Terms

recap

assist patients

base of support

malfunctioning equipment

tightly snap out

close to your body

overstuffing

spills

lowest position

work environment

call light

avoid jerky movements

unnecessary furniture

patients at risk

two-thirds full

push, pull or slide

trash room

squat

siderails

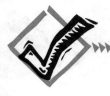

SAFETY MEASURES MATCH

ANSWER KEY

Needle Stick Prevention Safety Measures:

Never *recap* needles.
Empty sharps containers when *two-thirds full.*
Avoid *overstuffing* sharps containers.
Always *tightly snap* sharps container's lid upon disposal.
Place the full sharps container in the *trash room.*

Fall Prevention Safety Measures:

Assist patients at risk for falling with activities.
Return the bed to the *lowest position* after patient care.
Place the *call light* within the patient's reach.
Identify *patients at risk* for falls.
Raise *siderails* on beds when necessary.

Body Mechanics Safety Measures:

Squat instead of lifting whenever possible.
Stand with your feet apart to maintain a proper *base of support.*
When carrying objects hold them *close to your body.*
Push, pull or slide instead of bending to pick up heavy objects
    from the floor.
Avoid jerky movements when transferring patients.

Work Environment Safety Measures:

Wipe up *spills* immediately and call housekeeping if necessary.
Rolling equipment needs to be *out* of the hall.
Label *malfunctioning equipment* and notify appropriate
    department.
Remove *unnecessary furniture* and equipment from patient rooms.
Everyone is responsible for maintaining a safe *work environment.*

Safety Certificate

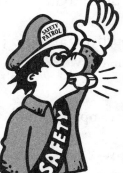

Safety Patrol Member

For participation in the Safety Exercise
as part of the
Annual Inservice Program

Instructor

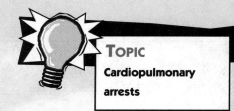

TOPIC
Cardiopulmonary arrests

TOOL BOX
Code crossword puzzle, pens or pencils, answer key

CODE CROSSWORD PUZZLE

Preparation

1. Copy as many ready-to-use Code crossword puzzles as there are participants.

2. Use the puzzle as an introduction to the lesson or as a review after the lesson.

3. Make sure each participant has a pen or pencil.

4. Make a copy of the answer key.

Variation

1. Use a poster printer copy machine to turn the crossword into a poster-size image.

2. Plan for groups of two to six to discuss and fill in a poster-size copy of the crossword puzzle before or after your lesson.

Implementation

1. Pass out the large or small crossword puzzle.

2. Challenge your learners to complete the puzzle as individuals or as teams.

3. If energy and attention are low during your lesson presentation, stop and let your participants engage in this energizing activity.

4. Crossword puzzles can also be sent out days or weeks after the lesson as reinforcement of important concepts.

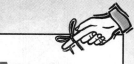

EDUCATOR SECRETS:
If you have different ability levels in your session, pair learners to maximize benefits to all.

By: Amanda Martin, MEd, BSN, RN, CNOR

CODE CROSSWORD PUZZLE

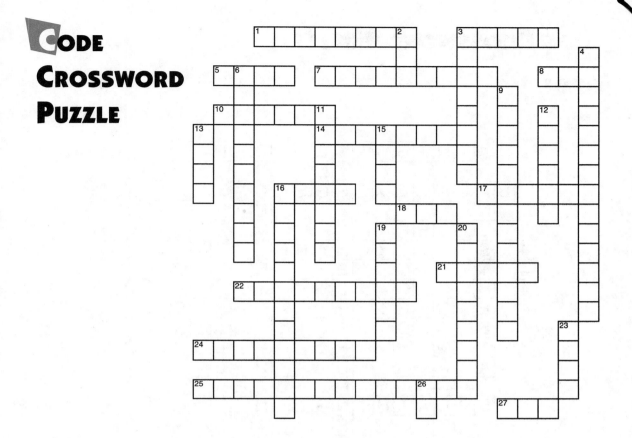

Across

1. A laryngoscope, blade, endo tube, and stylet are needed to do this
3. These are found in drawer 2 in the cart/pharmacy restocks these
5. The backboard is here on the Code cart
7. The _____ cord can be used to call for help; found in the bathroom
8. Masks with _____ shields are in drawer 4
10. The Team _____ runs the Code
14. What you do with the used cart after the code: _____ it with central supply department
16. This needs to be brought to the scene of the code immediately
17. A Code is a cardiac or respiratory _____
18. Number to call for Code at off-campus sites
21. To open the cart, you must do this to the lock
22. This is done through the mask found on the back of the door
24. The unit should STAT page the patient's _____ to notify him/her about the code
25. The _____ Coordinator attends every code and assists nursing
27. This should be initiated when someone is found pulseless and breathless

Down

2. The _____ Tech runs a continuous cardiac tracing of the code
3. Someone must _____ the events during the Code on the Code form
4. The laryngoscope, blade, and this should go to the head of the bed ASAP
6. The type of MD who comes to the code and intubates and maintains the airway
9. Used to "shock" patient and monitor heart's electrical activity
11. The nurse who documents the code signs as this on the Code form
12. A box of these should be on the front left cart to protect hands
13. The number used to call a code on the hospital campus
15. When someone codes, call for this
16. These are done using proper hand positioning on the patient's chest
19. A nursing assistant can be the _____ to get necessary items for the code
20. The excess _____ must be removed from the room so ACLS team can get in
23. Mouth to _____ is used to initiate artificial respirations
26. _____ access must be maintained to give drugs

15

CODE CROSSWORD PUZZLE

ANSWER KEY

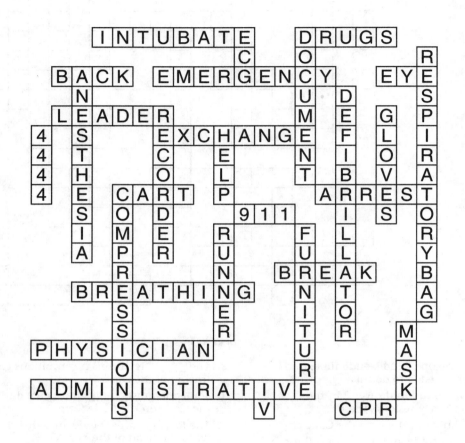

Across

1. Intubate
3. Drugs
5. Back
7. Emergency
8. Eye
10. Leader
14. Exchange
16. Cart
17. Arrest
18. 911
21. Break
22. Breathing
24. Physician
25. Administrative
27. CPR

Down

2. ECG
3. Document
4. Respiratory bag
6. Anesthesia
9. Defibrillator
11. Recorder
12. Gloves
13. 4444
15. Help
16. Compressions
19. Runner
20. Furniture
23. Mask
26. IV

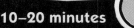
TOPIC

To quickly access and use the equipment in each drawer of the emergency cart in a code situation

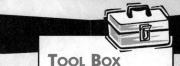

CODE CART CONTENTS CONTEST

Preparation

1. Calculate how many teams of two to five you will have.

2. Obtain a master list of the code cart contents in your institution. Make a copy of this for each team and use it as an answer key.

3. Obtain five envelopes per team.

4. Label the envelopes Drawer 1 through Drawer 5, or however many drawers your institution's code cart contains. Each team will need one set of the envelopes.

5. If necessary, adjust the Code Cart Contents Contest ready-to-use page so that it reflects your cart's contents. Make one copy per team.

6. Cut one copy of the ready-to-use page into sections along the black lines. This gives you forty-eight smaller sheets of paper. To assure that no sets get mixed up, write on the back of each of these pieces "set A." This will allow you to reuse the sets easily, even if they are mixed by the participants.

7. Randomly place the pieces in one set of the labeled envelopes.

8. Cut up the rest of the ready-to-use page copies as directed in steps 6 and 7. Label these "set B," "set C," and so forth.

9. Have a watch with a second hand or a stopwatch available for each team.

continued

TOOL BOX

For each team: 5 envelopes, set of words of cart's contents, answer key, watch with a second hand or timing device

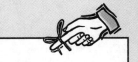

EDUCATOR SECRETS:

Encourage the teams by offering more than one opportunity to correctly categorize the items.

By: Amanda Martin, MEd, BSN, RN, CNOR

Code Cart Contents Contest *continued*

Implementation

1. Divide the learners into teams of two to five.

2. Supply each team with a set of labeled envelopes.

3. Direct the teams to empty their envelopes.

4. The team must examine all the paper strips and place them in the envelopes that correspond to the drawers that are on the cart. If an item does not belong in any drawer, they are to place it aside as a distractor. One person acts as team timer for the activity.

5. Hand out your institution's answer key. The group then consults the answer key to check themselves for accuracy.

6. The teams then rescramble all the pieces of paper. The answer key is placed out of sight.

7. The teams try again to locate the items as quickly as possible while one member times them.

8. Teams can compete against their first time to increase their speed and accuracy.

CODE CART CONTENTS CONTEST

Cart Contents for Categorizing

Alcohol/betadine swabs	Laryngoscope	Syringes
Miller/MacIntosh blades	Silk tape	Heparin
ECG leads & paper	McGill forceps	Narcan
Regular & spinal needles	Dextrose 50%	Filter straws
Atropine bristoject	Epinephrine	Blood set
Pre-mix lidocaine	Pre-mix dopamine	Jelcos
Intraosseous needles	Armboards	Microdrip tubing
1000cc sodium chloride	Buretrols	Extension sets 35"
Catheterization tray	Gloves, gowns	4 x 4s
Ambu foot suction pump	Salem sump kit	Masks/eyeshields
Blood pressure cuffs	Introducer kit	Endotracheal tubes
Adult respiratory bag	Stylets	Oxygen tubing
Pediatric respiratory bag	Airways	Ambu w/reservoir
Blood gas syringes	Glucagon	Digoxin
IVAC tubing	Pacemaker	Skin prep pads
Hydrogen peroxide	Saline pads	Ammonia ampules

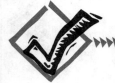

CODE CART CONTENTS CONTEST

Directions: Sample answer key for cart content papers. Obtain your institution's list, which might differ from this one.

Drawer 1
Syringes
Laryngoscope
Miller/MacIntosh blades
Silk tape
ECG leads & paper
Alcohol/betadine swabs
Regular & spinal needles
McGill forceps

Drawer 2
Filter straws
Atropine bristoject
Pre-mix lidocaine
Pre-mix dopamine
Epinephrine
Heparin
Narcan
Dextrose 50%

Drawer 3
Intraosseous needles
Armboards
Blood set
Microdrip tubing
Jelcos
1000cc sodium chloride
Buretrols
Extension sets 35"

Drawer 4
4 x 4s
Gloves, gowns
Catheterization tray
Salem sump kit
Ambu foot suction pump
Masks/eyeshields
Introducer kit
Blood pressure cuffs

Drawer 5
Adult respiratory bag
Pediatric respiratory bag
Stylets
Endotracheal tubes
Ambu w/reservoir
Oxygen tubing
Airways
Blood gas syringes

Distractors
Glucagon
Digoxin
IVAC tubing
Pacemaker
Skin prep pads
Hydrogen peroxide
Saline pads
Ammonia ampules

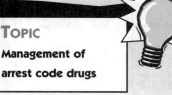
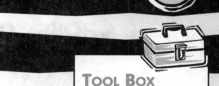

TOOL BOX
Management of
Arrest Code Drugs
crossword puzzle,
pens or pencils,
answer key

MANAGEMENT OF ARREST CODE DRUGS CROSSWORD PUZZLE

Preparation

1. Make a copy of the ready-to-use Management of Arrest Code Drugs crossword puzzle for each participant.
2. Use this as an introduction to the lesson or as a review after the lesson.
3. Make sure each participant has a pen or pencil.
4. Make a copy of the answer key.

Variation

1. Use a poster printer copy machine to turn the crossword into a poster-size image.
2. Plan for groups of two to six to discuss and fill in a poster-size copy of the crossword puzzle before or after your lesson.

Implementation

1. Pass out the large or small crossword puzzle.
2. Challenge your learners to complete the puzzle as individuals or as teams.
3. If energy and attention are low during your lesson presentation, stop and let your participants engage in this energizing activity.
4. Crossword puzzles can also be sent out days or weeks after the lesson as reinforcement of important concepts.

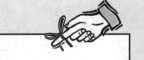

EDUCATOR
SECRETS:

If you have different
ability levels in your
session, pair learners
to maximize benefits
to all.

By: Amanda Martin, MEd,
BSN, RN, CNOR

MANAGEMENT OF ARREST CODE DRUGS CROSSWORD PUZZLE

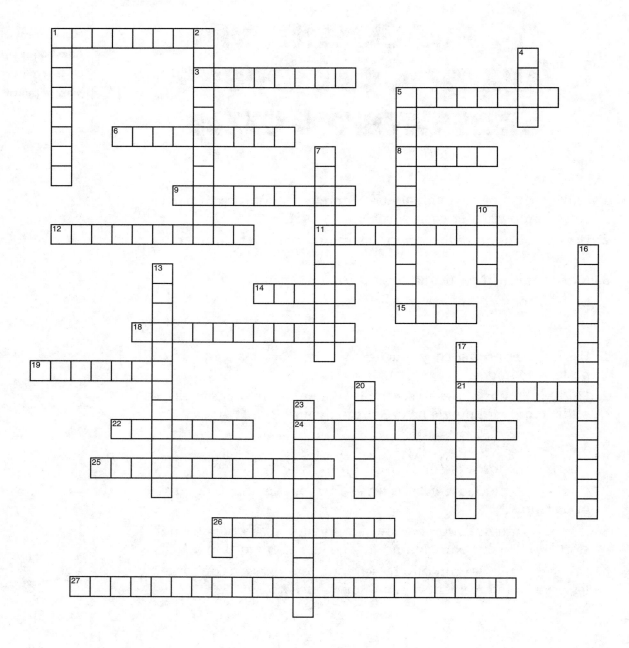

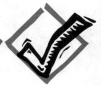

MANAGEMENT OF ARREST CODE DRUGS CROSSWORD PUZZLE

Across

1. Drug of choice to treat bradycardia
3. Increases cardiac output, urine output, and BP
5. Indicated for insulin shock
6. Used to treat supraventricular tachycardias
8. Slang for defibrillation
9. First line drug for ventricular arrhythmias
11. Bretylium is used for recurrent or _____ ventricular arrhythmias
12. Term used to describe code drug "syringe"
14. This is followed by a drip for drugs like lidocaine and procainamide
15. Treatment of choice for sinus rhythm
18. Synonym for dysrhythmias
19. Used to treat asystole or third degree heart block
21. This needs to be done to the cardiac rhythm to determine which drugs to use
22. Term used to describe adjusting drip to patient's response to the drug
24. Route of administration of most code drugs
25. This tube is used for airway maintenance and may be used to administer epinephrine and atropine
26. The type of tubing used to administer code drugs via drip
27. This cardiac rhythm may be sustained or degenerate into ventricular fibrillation

Down

1. Epinephrine is the first line drug for this; absence of a cardiac rhythm
2. This drug increases heart rate, automaticity, myocardial contractility
4. Most code drugs are given by this method
5. Electromechanical _____
7. Lidocaine, bretylium, and procainamide are used to treat these arrhythmias
10. Dopamine is given *only* by this method
13. Defibrillation is the treatment of choice for ventricular _____
16. Furosemide is indicated for this condition
17. This is a severe complication of intracardiac administration of drugs
20. Narcotic antagonist
23. Sodium _____ is given to reverse metabolic acidosis; *not* a first line drug
26. Unit of measure for most drugs

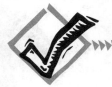

MANAGEMENT OF ARREST CODE DRUGS CROSSWORD PUZZLE

ANSWER KEY

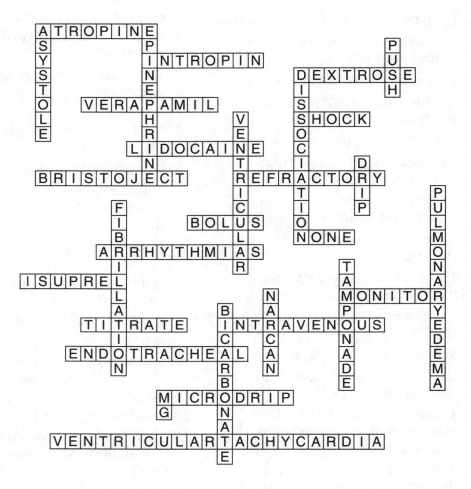

Across

1. Atropine
3. Intropin
5. Dextrose
6. Verapamil
8. Shock
9. Lidocaine
11. Refractory
12. Bristoject
14. Bolus
15. None
18. Arrhythmias
19. Isuprel
21. Monitor

22. Titrate
24. Intravenous
25. Endotracheal
26. Microdrip
27. Ventricular tachycardia

Down

1. Asystole
2. Epinephrine
4. Push
5. Dissociation
7. Ventricular
10. Drip
13. Fibrillation
16. Pulmonary edema
17. Tamponade
20. Narcan
23. Bicarbonate
26. mg

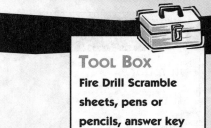

FIRE DRILL SCRAMBLE

Preparation

1. Read the Fire Drill Scramble answer key to make sure that this information agrees with your institution's procedures on how to handle fires.

2. Add, delete, or change any necessary items on both ready-to-use pages so that they fit your individual needs.

3. Copy enough Fire Drill Scramble sheets and answer keys so that each participant will have one.

4. Make sure each participant has a pen or pencil.

Implementation

1. Have your learners first unscramble the words alone or as a team.

2. Ask them to fill in the blanks with an appropriate unscrambled answer.

3. Inform learners that there are more answers than there are blanks and that answers can be used only once.

4. After the game, clarify and discuss any confusing issues.

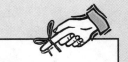

By: Nancy Hennen, BSN, RNC

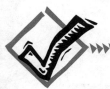

FIRE DRILL SCRAMBLE

Directions: The following exercise is a review of fire drills. Fill in the blanks with the appropriate unscrambled answer. There are more scrambled answers than there are blanks.

1. The evacuation routes for the hospital are usually the stairs. If these routes are not available, the _____ is used.

2. It is important to make sure that all the _____ on the unit are closed.

3. A _____ fire extinguisher is used for trash can fires.

4. When first calling the switchboard, you need to tell the operator your name, location, and extension number. You then _____ up the phone.

5. The _____ will call you back and then you tell her or him the location, the type, and the extent of the fire.

6. You need to _____ the door before entering a room where there may be a fire.

7. The correct way to use a fire extinguisher is with a _____ motion.

8. The CO_2 extinguisher is located in the _____.

9. One hundred twenty (120) chimes/minute indicates a _____-stage alarm.

10. Twenty (20) chimes/minute indicates a _____-stage alarm.

FIRE DRILL SCRAMBLE

ANSWER KEY

Key Terms

ptoreaor (operator)

stifr (first)

twes [*distractor*]

sorod (doors)

cektnih (kitchen)

lnicci (clinic)

$_2$OC [*distractor*]

tware (water)

sate [*distractor*]

descon (second)

tnohr [*distractor*]

hdirt [*distractor*]

elef (feel)

ghna (hang)

desi ot esdi
  (side to side)

eplen [*distractor*]

1. The evacuation routes for the hospital are usually the stairs. If these routes are not available, the _____clinic_____ is used.

2. It is important to make sure that all the _____doors_____ on the unit are closed.

3. A _____water_____ fire extinguisher is used for trash can fires.

4. When first calling the switchboard, you need to tell the operator your name, location, and extension number. You then _____hang_____ up the phone.

5. The _____operator_____ will call you back and then you tell her or him the location, the type, and the extent of the fire.

6. You need to _____feel_____ the door before entering a room where there may be a fire.

7. The correct way to use a fire extinguisher is with a _____side to side_____ motion.

8. The CO_2 extinguisher is located in the _____kitchen_____.

9. One hundred twenty (120) chimes/minute indicates a _____second_____-stage alarm.

10. Twenty (20) chimes/minute indicates a _____first_____-stage alarm.

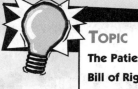

TOOL BOX

Questions, buzzing device, small rewards, answer key

WHAT'S RIGHT WITH RIGHTS?

Preparation

1. Make a copy of the *What's Right with Rights?* Questions and Answers ready-to-use page.

2. Obtain a buzzing device and small rewards.

Implementation

1. Explain to the group that they will be asked nine questions regarding the Patient's Bill of Rights.

2. Divide the group into teams to answer the questions.

3. Read each question aloud to the participants.

4. The participants compete as teams to answer the questions.

5. The first team to "buzz in" may answer the question.

6. Rewards are given for each question or for the highest total number of correct responses.

7. Use this game to foster discussion and clarify information.

EDUCATOR SECRETS:

Try to equalize competition between groups.

By: Michele Deck, MEd, BSN, RN, ACCE-R
Nancy Hennen, BSN, RNC

WHAT'S RIGHT WITH RIGHTS?

QUESTIONS

1. The nurse asks you to put 548 on the bedpan. What's wrong with this?

2. A new patient is admitted to the unit. You see that his name is listed as John Downs. You enter the room to answer the call light. You begin talking to him. How do you know what name to call him?

3. You enter a patient's room. You tell him that he is going for a UGI and you need to get him a gown for it. He has a puzzled look on his face. What should you do?

4. A patient who is paraplegic asks you, "Will I ever be able to move my legs again?" What do you say?

5. You go into the room to turn the patient in bed. She says, "Don't touch me. I just got comfortable." Do you turn the patient anyway?

6. You are in the elevator, and two people behind you are discussing Mrs. Bounds, a difficult patient on their unit. What's wrong with this conversation?

7. You are going to catheterize a patient. The curtains on the window are open, and the door to the hall is slightly open. What needs to be done to ensure the patient's privacy?

8. You have been assigned a patient who asks if her grandchild can come visit. What do you say?

9. You walk into a patient's room for the first time on your shift. You say to her, "Hello, my name is Nancy, and I'm your nursing care technician for today." Your name tag is visible, and the patient looks at it and says, "Oh, yes, Nancy. I am Mrs. Bounds. What are you going to do to me today?" What do you say?

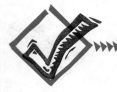

WHAT'S RIGHT WITH RIGHTS?

ANSWER KEY

1. The patient has the right to be treated as a person, not as a room number.

2. Always ask the patient what name you should call him or her. Some people are uncomfortable being called by their first name. Some do not like being called "Honey" or "Sweetie" or similar names.

3. The patient has the right to information in a form that he or she can understand. Unfamiliar words or abbreviations shouldn't be used. Explain in simple terms that a UGI is an X-ray.

4. If at any time a patient asks you a question about his or her condition, refer the patient to the nurse or doctor in charge.

5. If the patient refuses treatment, do not force him or her. Report to the nurse what the patient said.

6. Information about patients is never discussed in public areas. You should only discuss patient information with the nurse with whom you are working.

7. Pull the curtains on the window, pull the privacy curtain, and shut the door. Always make sure that the patient is covered, exposing only the part of the body that is needed for treatment.

8. Patients need to know the hospitals visiting hours and policy. The patient has a right to know what the rules are.

9. There is nothing wrong with this scenario. To reinterate: Always introduce yourself with your name, title, and always wear your name tag. All staff members may look the same to the patient.

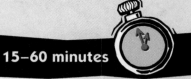
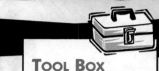
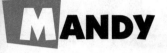

MANDY

TOOL BOX
Mandy bingo sheets,
Mandy question
cards, pens or
pencils, small
goodies or prizes

Preparation

1. Write questions on your annual mandatory review topic on 3" x 5" cards.

2. Write the one or two word answers (instead of numbers) in the squares on sheets resembling bingo cards. (See sample on the next page.)

3. Write the word MANDY instead of BINGO on top of the sheet. The answers must be in different squares on each sheet, or there must be different answers on each sheet.

4. Copy enough Mandy cards so that each participant will have one.

5. Obtain small prizes or goodies for giveaways.

6. Make sure each participant has a pen or pencil.

Implementation

1. Explain to the group that this game is played like Bingo. Participants are to mark off the correct answers as they are called. The first person with squares marked off in a row vertically, horizontally, or diagonally must yell, "Mandy!"

2. Shuffle and cut the 3" x 5" cards and begin to ask the questions.

3. If the holder of the Mandy sheet has the answer, that square is marked. The game proceeds as in Bingo.

4. When someone yells, "Mandy," check their card and award a small prize.

5. Play enough games so that all questions have been read.

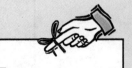

EDUCATOR SECRETS:
Play "blackout
Mandy" and require
that participants
completely cover
their cards to win as
in "blackout bingo."

By: Miriam Sheridan, EdD,
    MN, RN

MANDY

M	A	N	D	Y
Tongue	Gown and Gloves	Gloves	Extinguish Fire	Recapping
Puncture Resistant Container	Are You Choking?	Show of Force	Radiation Safety Officer	Hazard Warning Label
5 to 1	Activate Alarm	**FREE**	Key	Informed Consent
Blood and Body Fluid	q TOD	RN	Advance Directives	MSDS
5911	Remove Occupants	Eating	CPR	Body Mechanics

EXAMPLE QUESTIONS

Under "M"

1. The most common cause of airway obstruction in the unconscious victim is the _____.

2. After use, needles should not be recapped but placed in a _____.

3. The ratio of compressions to ventilations in a two-rescuer CPR is _____.

4. Major infections hazards particularly with AIDS are _____.

5. The phone extension number for calling a code is _____.

DOCUMENTING CODE BLUE

... Without One Happening

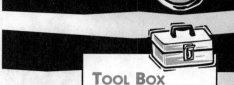

25–30 minutes

TOOL BOX

Videocamera,
code documentation
sheets, watch for
each participant,
overhead of blank
sheet, overhead of
completed sheet
for review, pens or
pencils

Preparation

1. If a code team responds to arrest within your hospital, the staff nurses may act as recorders. If these staff people are nervous on a daily basis about the task of "recorder," this exercise may help.

2. Get some of the emergency room staff, life flight crew, and respiratory care department together to do a mock code video for the nursing education staff.

3. Choose any kind of scenario that is typical for your facility. A sample scenario appears on the ready-to-use page.

4. Copy the scenario and give it out to each actor. In the background out of camera range, you might include a white board with the script attached for the actors. A manikin is used as the patient.

5. Set up a video camera in the corner of the room so that it can record all of the code activities. (Some people use personal video cameras; others use their institution's equipment.)

6. Film the scenario. Make it about twelve minutes long. Watch it to see if it needs restaging.

7. Gather your institution's code documentation sheet and make an overhead of it. Copy enough code documentation sheets so that each learner can have at least one.

8. Make sure each participant has a pen or pencil.

Implementation

1. Review the code documentation sheet with handouts and overhead, answering any questions learners may have.

2. Show the video. Have the group use their watch and code documentation sheets to document the events they are witnessing on the video.

3. Review the video and show an overhead completely filled out.

4. Answer any questions and concerns the learners may have regarding the process.

5. The video and worksheets can be loaned out to those who need more practice.

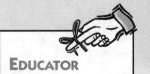

EDUCATOR SECRETS:

The participants
appreciate the
practice before
the real thing.

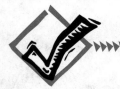

DOCUMENTING CODE BLUE

. . . Without One Happening

SAMPLE CODE SCENARIO

A middle-aged woman who was admitted the day before with shortness of breath is unresponsive when the caregiver comes in to check vital signs. The code response is initiated, and the team arrives (ER physician, nurses, respiratory therapist), and the code proceeds per ACLS standards.

TOPIC

Required annual
reviews or any type
of dry or lengthy
content

HOSPITAL TIC TAC TOE

TOOL BOX

9 cards with an *X*
on one side and
an *O* on the other,
3 chairs, prizes,
questions to ask

Preparation

1. Develop fifty multiple-choice or true/false questions from JCAHO and OSHA mandatory review requirements for personnel.

2. Prepare nine 8 1/2" x 11" cardboard playing pieces. Place an *X* on one side of the pieces and an *O* on the other.

3. Place three chairs in a row in the front of the room.

4. Consult the attendance list to see if there are nine people who are not shy and would want to come up front as a "star" or "contestant."

5. Obtain some small prizes or goodies for all who participate.

Implementation

1. As participants come in for the program, nine people are recruited to be stars. Arrange the nine people so that three sit in the chairs, three stand behind the chairs, and three sit on the floor in front of the chairs.

2. Each star receives a cardboard playing piece.

3. Divide the audience into two teams, the *X*s and the *O*s.

4. Pick a spokesperson for each team. They will act as contestants. The facilitator and the two contestants stand in the front of the room looking at the participants.

5. Explain to the team that the object of the game is to score three *X*s or *O*s in a row either horizontally, vertically, or diagonally.

6. Each team will take a turn picking a square.

7. The facilitator reads a question to the star in that square, giving him or her a true/false or multiple-choice question.

continued

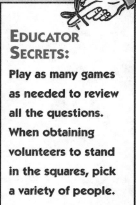

EDUCATOR
SECRETS:

Play as many games
as needed to review
all the questions.
When obtaining
volunteers to stand
in the squares, pick
a variety of people.

By: Nancy Wilson, MSN, RN

HOSPITAL TIC TAC TOE   *continued*

8. The star in the square announces his or her answer to the audience.

9. The team's spokesperson indicates if the team believes the star's answer is correct or not.

10. The facilitator reveals the correct answer.

11. Teams win squares by *correctly* agreeing or *correctly* disagreeing with the star. The star then displays the appropriate *X* or *O* side of the cardboard playing piece.

12. Explain to the stars ahead of time that they do not have to know the answers, just act like they do!

13. The team that wins the most games receives a small prize, usually candy. The nine stars also receive a goodie.

HOSPITAL TIC TAC TOE

SAMPLE QUESTIONS

Directions: Both true/false and multiple choice questions can be used during this game since the team's responsibility is to agree or disagree with the star. With multiple-choice questions, the star picks the answer after the facilitator reads the questions.

Here are some sample questions to get you started:

True/False

1. Restraints may be used for punishment.
2. One of the goals of risk management is to identify and control risk and reduce liability.
3. The AIDS virus can live outside the body for prolonged periods of time.

Multiple Choice

4. If a fire cannot be extinguished with a fire extinguisher, you should

   a. open the doors and windows so the smoke and fire can escape.
   b. close the door to the room where the fire is located.
   c. prop the door halfway open so you can keep an eye on the smoke and flames.

5. During a tornado alert, nonambulatory patients should

   a. not be moved.
   b. be put under the beds.
   c. be moved away from windows and covered with blankets.
   d. have an IV of D5W started.

6. What does MSDS stand for?

   a. Micro Surgical Dose Standards
   b. Materially Serious Dangerous Substances
   c. Material Safety Data Sheets

7. What does the *UL* in UL Approved stand for?

   a. Underwires Limited
   b. Unlicensed Lectricians
   c. Underwriters Laboratory

8. In the acronym RACE, the *C* stands for:

   a. call the fire department
   b. carry out the patients
   c. close the doors
   d. cry

9. The announcement of a CODE RED means:

   a. a fire drill
   b. a patient has arrested
   c. Santa has been spotted on the roof
   d. the area noted with the code should be evacuated

TOPIC
Orientation for new employees to the physical layout of the facility.

TOOL BOX
Photo negative made into a puzzle, ziplock bags, transparent tape, note cards, map of your institution

PUZZLING SCAVENGER HUNT

Preparation

1. Take a photo of something meaningful at your institution (a statue, a logo, or new equipment).

2. Have an 8" x 10" photo negative made into a puzzle approximately 8" x 10" in size. If this service is unavailable to you, have an 8" x 10" print made and cut it into pieces.

3. Divide the puzzle pieces equally into four to six ziplock bags.

4. Place a note card in each bag giving a clue as to where the next piece will be located.

5. Place these at different locations as indicated by your clues.

6. Make a map of your institution and copy it so that each participant has one.

Implementation

1. Invite the group of orientees to find the places and the puzzle pieces.

2. Distribute the maps. Give the group the first clue.

3. During and after lunch the group can put the puzzle together to discover the important photo displayed.

4. Ask the group to summarize their journey in a three-minute discussion.

EDUCATOR SECRETS:
If some of the orientees know the layout, have them spend 1–2 minutes discussing the area with the new people on the tour.

By: Theresa Rimer, BSN, RN, CPN

TOPIC

Basic Life Support
review for any
content that has
questions and
answers.

20 minutes

TOOL BOX

Play money,
multicolored party
balloons (4 colors)
containing pieces of
paper with questions

BALLOON BURST RELAY

Preparation

1. Write at least twenty commonly asked questions about Basic
   Life Support on small pieces of paper.
2. Divide the questions by level of difficulty into four categories.
3. Obtain four differently colored balloons. Place the questions of
   the same difficulty inside the same colored balloons, placing one
   question in each balloon.
4. Blow up the balloons and tie them.
5. Keep a master list of questions and answers for reference.
6. Use play money for prizes.

Variation

1. Use an answer given, question asked format. Red balloons have
   $1000 answers; green, $500; blue, $100; pink $50.

Implementation

1. Explain that the purpose of this activity is to review CPR theory
   and skills in a fun way.
2. Divide the group into two teams.
3. In front of the class, position two chairs and a variety of balloons.
4. Explain that the color coding relates to the level of difficulty
   of the questions.

continued

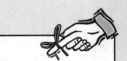

EDUCATOR SECRETS:

The class is prepared
for the written test
at the end of game.

By: Gretchen Hrachovec,
MA, BSN, RNC

BALLOON BURST RELAY *continued*

5. On a signal from the scorekeeper, one person from each team races to the front of the room, grabs a balloon, and sits on it to break it. Whoever breaks a balloon first wins $25 (play money) for the team and answers the question in the balloon. If the answer is correct, an additional $25 is awarded.

6. If the person cannot answer the question, the balloon breaker of the opposite team gets a crack at it.

7. All *money* earned by individuals goes to their team.

8. Color coding the balloons according to the difficulty of the questions (and the chance to earn more money) excites competitors and avoids the embarrassment that might occur if a person has not reviewed BLS before going to class.

9. The little papers with the questions can be reused for the next class.

TOPIC

Adult and/or child Heimlich maneuver. Jingles and raps can be used to reinforce important concepts.

5–10 minutes

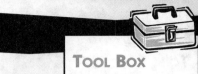

TOOL BOX

CPR manikin for practice, words to the "Heimlich Hokey Pokey" song

HEIMLICH HOKEY POKEY

Preparation

1. Set up your CPR class materials and supplies.
2. Practice the "Heimlich Hokey Pokey" song or have a written copy with you.

Implementation

1. Explain the steps of adult and/or child obstructive airway rescue.
2. Demonstrate the proper hand placement.
3. Teach the group the song "Heimlich Hokey Pokey."
4. Have the group practice the procedure while singing the "Heimlich Hokey Pokey":

    You put your right fist in,

    You keep your thumb side out.

    You put your left hand on,

    And you're lifting in and up.

    You do the Heimlich Hokey Pokey,

    And you clear the airway out.

    That's what it's all about.

5. Have the class practice and demonstrate their skills to the CPR instructor.
6. Proceed with CPR skills checkoff.

EDUCATOR SECRETS:

It doesn't matter if you can sing or not. Think of the alphabet song!

By: Jann Christensen, MPA, BSN, RN

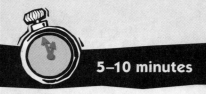

TOOL BOX
One set of cards in an envelope for each team

BUSY BODIES

Preparation

1. Make two copies of the Busy Bodies ready-to-use sheet.
2. Cut both sheets along the black lines dividing the information.
3. Place each set of strips in an envelope.
4. If you have a large group, make a set for each team of two to six people.

Implementation

1. Divide the participants into two groups.
2. Each group receives a complete set of strips.
3. Explain that the goal is to choose the correct body mechanics statements, eliminating the strips with the incorrect statements.
4. When this is done, one team begins by explaining its choice of strips, then the other explains its choice.
5. Finish up by discussing pertinent points that need clarification and reinforcement.

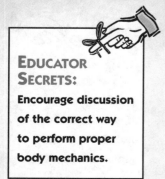

EDUCATOR SECRETS:
Encourage discussion of the correct way to perform proper body mechanics.

**By: Michele Deck, MEd, BSN, RN, ACCE-R
Nancy Hennen, BSN, RNC**

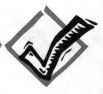

Busy Bodies

Directions: Copy these and cut for one card set.

Never twist to reach an object.	Never lift heavy patients without help.
Always squat to lift heavy objects.	Avoid sudden jerky movements.
Always use both hands.	Hold heavy objects with one hand.
Avoid unnecessary bending and reaching.	Bring the bed to the lowest position to make it.
Push, slide, or roll objects whenever possible.	Always bend from the waist.
Make sure that your body is in good alignment and that you have a wide base of support.	Hold objects that you are carrying as far away from your body as possible.
Stand close to the object to be lifted.	

43

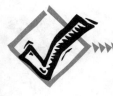

BUSY BODIES

ANSWER KEY

Busy Bodies cards contain one of each of the statements below.

Correct

Never twist to reach an object.

Always squat to lift heavy objects.

Always use both hands.

Avoid unnecessary bending and reaching.

Push, slide, or roll objects whenever possible.

Make sure that your body is in good alignment
and that you have a wide base of support.

Stand close to the object to be lifted.

Never lift heavy patients without help.

Avoid sudden jerky movements.

Incorrect

Hold heavy objects with one hand.

Bring the bed to the lowest position to make it.

Always bend from the waist.

Hold objects that you are carrying as far away
from your body as possible.

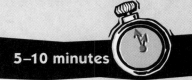
ASEPTIC RE-VIEW

Preparation

1. Enlarge the Aseptic Re-View ready-to-use windowpane picture, so that when displayed the windowpane pictures can be seen and identified by each person in the room.

2. Have the Aseptic Re-View ready-to-use picture answer key on hand for your use.

Implementation

1. Explain to your learners that you are using each picture as a visual cue for each of the eight concepts to be remembered.

2. Begin in the top left corner of the windowpane and explain that the first principle of asepsis is that "all items used in a sterile field must be sterile." The way to ensure that an item is sterile is to observe that the package is intact, just as this "package" is wrapped and untorn.

3. Next, move to the top right-hand corner of the windowpane. Explain that the second principle is "a sterile barrier that is torn or wet is not sterile." This picture represents a torn package with water dripping over it.

4. Continue to move down and across the windowpanes discussing each principle and how the picture represents the principle.

5. At the end of the explanation, simply begin at the top corner and point to each picture. Let the students recall each principle based on the picture they see.

6. Leave the content for a time and come back to the pictures to review.

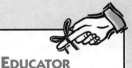

EDUCATOR SECRETS:
A majority of learners are visual and remember the pictures clearly.

By: Michele Deck, MEd, BSN, RN, ACCE-R
Nancy Hennen, BSN, RNC

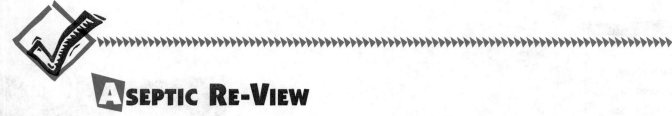

ASEPTIC RE-VIEW

WINDOWPANE

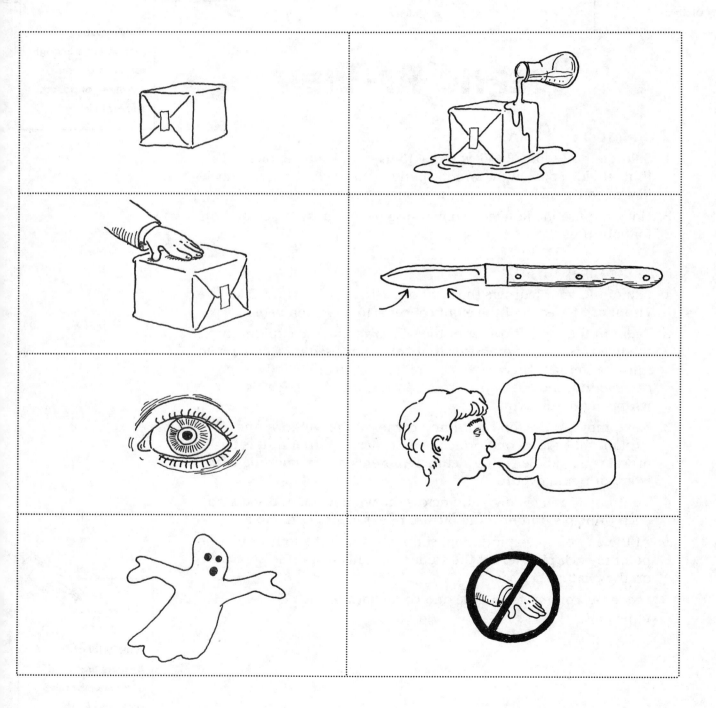

Copyright © 1995 by Mosby–Year Book, Inc.

ASEPTIC RE-VIEW

ANSWER KEY

All items used in a sterile field must be sterile. (Make sure the package is intact.)	A sterile barrier that is torn or wet is not sterile.
Never touch the inside of a sterile package with your hands.	The edges of a sterile container are unsterile once they are open.
It is only sterile if you can see it.	Never cough, sneeze, or talk over a sterile field.
Never reach across a sterile field.	Once you touch a patient with an object, it is no longer sterile.

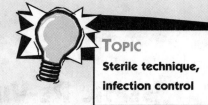

TOOL BOX
Septic Secrets
crossword puzzle,
pens or pencils,
answer key

SEPTIC SECRETS CROSSWORD PUZZLE

Preparation

1. Copy the ready-to-use Septic Secrets crossword puzzle, making sure you have one copy per participant.

2. Use this as an introduction to the lesson or as a review after the lesson.

3. Make sure each participant has a pen or pencil.

4. Make a copy of the answer key.

Variation

1. Use a poster printer copy machine to turn the crossword into a poster-size image.

2. Plan for groups of two to six to discuss and fill in a poster-size copy of the crossword puzzle before or after your lesson.

Implementation

1. Pass out the large or small crossword puzzle.

2. Challenge your learners to complete the puzzle as individuals or as teams.

3. If energy and attention are low during your lesson presentation, stop and let your participants engage in this energizing activity.

4. Crossword puzzles can also be sent out days or weeks after the lesson as reinforcement of important concepts.

EDUCATOR SECRETS:
If you have different experience levels in your session, pair learners to maximize benefits to all.

By: Nancy Hennen, BSN, RNC

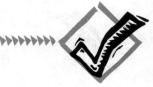

SEPTIC SECRETS CROSSWORD PUZZLE

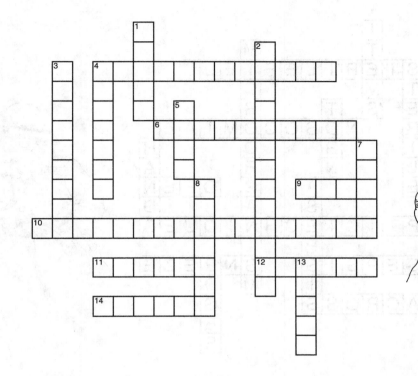

Across

4. An area that is free of all microorganisms
6. Hospital acquired
9. The edges of a sterile container are unsterile once they are _____
10. Practice that eliminates infectious pathogens from a work area
11. Infection
12. Never cough, _____, or talk over a sterile field
14. Never reach _____ a sterile field

Down

1. All _____ used in a sterile field must be sterile
2. Tiny forms of life that you are unable to see without a microscope
3. Any disease producing microorganisms
4. Free of all microorganisms
5. A sterile barrier that is wet or _____ is not sterile
7. Never touch the inside of a sterile package with your bare _____
8. Without infection
13. The _____ of a sterile container are unsterile once they are open

SEPTIC SECRETS CROSSWORD PUZZLE

ANSWER KEY

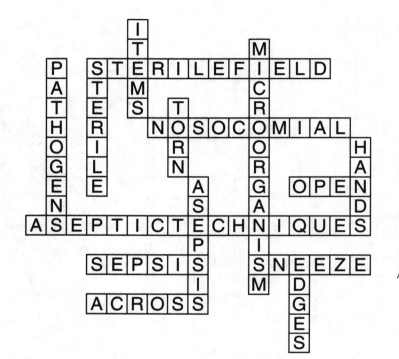

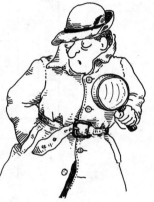

Across

4. sterile
6. nosocomial
9. open
10. aseptic techniques
11. sepsis
12. sneeze
14. across

Down

1. items
2. microorganism
3. pathogens
4. sterile
5. torn
7. hands
8. asepsis
13. edges

CRASH CART TREASURE HUNT

Preparation

1. Copy the ready-to-use Crash Cart Treasure Hunt page.
2. Cut the sheet on the lines dividing the clues.
3. Fold the clue sheets in half or in fourths.
4. Copy the answer key.
5. Make a note that reads, "Congratulations! You've reached the end of the hunt!"
6. Prepare your fully stocked code cart by placing Clue #2 on or beside the electrodes.
7. Place Clue #3 on or beside the code cart documentation or flow sheet.
8. Place Clue #4 on or beside the tourniquet.
9. Place Clue #5 on or beside the atropine.
10. Place Clue #6 on or beside the intubation supplies or box.
11. Place Clue #7 on or beside the introducer set.
12. Place Clue #8 on or beside the N/G tubes.
13. Place Clue # 9 on or beside the IV tubing.
14. Place a note on or beside the blood pressure cuff that says, "Congratulations! You've reached the end of the hunt!"

Implementation

1. Explain that this is a quick way for participants to explore the crash cart. The object is to go through all drawers and/or shelves during the treasure hunt.
2. Read the first clue aloud to the group. The clue leads the participants to the first item in the crash cart.
3. Tell them to follow the clues as a team.
4. The treasure hunt is complete when all clues and items have been found.
5. Celebrate with your learners by cheering with them. Give them positive verbal reinforcement.
6. Clarify and discuss any questions.

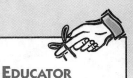

By: Susan B. Roders, BSN, RN

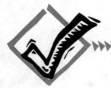

CRASH CART TREASURE HUNT

CLUE CARDS

Clue #1   I'm stuck on the body to get an ECG tracing.
           Now you can see if the heart is racing.

Clue #2   Now the code team is on the go.
           Someone better write down the flow.

Clue #3   An IV is needed! An IV is needed!
           I am used so the blood flow will be impeded.

Clue #4   The heart rate is a little slow.
           I'm given to give the heart some get up and go.

Clue #5   Now it's time to do the intubation.
           What supplies should I grab? What a tense situation!

Clue #6   A peripheral line is difficult to find.
           Now the doctor decides to insert central lines.

Clue #7   The patient's stomach is starting to inflate.
           Put an N/G tube down, and don't be late.

Clue #8   The IV is in, and you need to make the connection.
           Keep the end of this item sterile; we don't want an infection.

Clue #9   Now the patient's heart is beating.
           I am used to see what blood pressure we might be treating.

CRASH CART TREASURE HUNT

ANSWER KEY

Clue #1	I'm stuck on the body to get an ECG tracing.
	Now you can see if the heart is racing.
	(Electrodes)

Clue #2	Now the code team is on the go.
	Someone better write down the flow.
	(Code cart flow sheet)

Clue #3	An IV is needed! An IV is needed!
	I am used so the blood flow will be impeded.
	(Tourniquet)

Clue #4	The heart rate is a little slow.
	I'm given to give the heart some get up and go.
	(Atropine)

Clue #5	Now it's time to do the intubation.
	What supplies should I grab? What a tense situation!
	(Intubation box)

Clue #6	A peripheral line is difficult to find.
	Now the doctor decides to insert central lines.
	(Introducer set)

Clue #7	The patient's stomach is starting to inflate.
	Put an N/G tube down, and don't be late.
	(N/G tube)

Clue #8	The IV is in, and you need to make the connection.
	Keep the end of this item sterile; we don't want an infection.
	(IV tubing)

Clue #9	Now the patient's heart is beating. I am used to see what
	blood pressure we might be treating.
	(Blood pressure cuff)

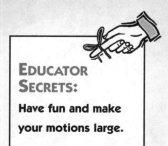

TOOL BOX

CPR manikins and regular supplies for recertification course

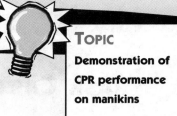
MIME CPR

Preparation

1. Review the steps of CPR performance before you begin your session.

Implementation

When performing recertifications for CPR, instead of doing a passive watch and listen, make it interactive, get the participants involved.

1. Explain that you will demonstrate silently the proper sequence of steps but that it is their job to say aloud and in unison the step being performed.

2. Mimic each step in sequence pausing momentarily for the learners to shout the step you are performing. For example, you shake the manikin. The group responds, "Determine unresponsiveness!"

3. Continue each step with learners saying aloud the proper sequence before they must return demonstrate.

4. Continue until sequence is finished.

5. Encourage everyone to clap or cheer to congratulate themselves and to build confidence before they perform.

EDUCATOR SECRETS:

Have fun and make your motions large.

By: Michele Deck, MEd, BSN, RN, ACCE-R

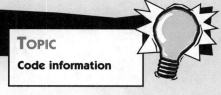

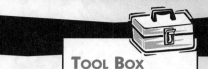

Code Questions, Not Answers

Preparation

1. Review the information on the ready-to-use Code Questions, Not Answers answer key. If it does not agree with your institution's policies, procedures, and information, edit it.

2. Make an overhead transparency from the ready-to-use amount and category sheet. A poster can also be used.

3. Copy the answer key to use when the learners pick a category and an amount.

4. Copy the questions for answers sheet, and use it to check the learners' responses.

5. Obtain a buzzing device.

6. Place a Post-it™ note on the transparency of the category and amount sheet after a square is chosen.

7. Collect small prizes or goodies (fruit, Post-it™ notes, etc.) to use as awards.

continued

By: Amanda Martin, MEd, BSN, RN, CNOR

CODE QUESTIONS, NOT ANSWERS *continued*

Implementation

1. Divide the group into two or more teams of three to six learners.

2. Explain that the teams may collaborate on the questions.

3. Pick a team to go first. Display the playing board on the overhead projector. A spokesperson for the team selects a category and an amount.

4. The instructor reads the answer from that category and amount.

5. Teams compete to be recognized with a buzzer system.

6. The teams can discuss their ideas quietly for up to five seconds before answering.

7. A team spokesperson states the question that fits the answer the instructor has given.

8. If the question given is correct, the team is awarded points based on how much their question is worth. If the answer is incorrect, the instructor can give the other team a chance to answer, or simply reveal the correct answer.

9. Points are tallied for each team.

10. After all answers are given, the team with the most points wins.

11. Award prizes to all participants. Because their knowledge has increased, they are all winners.

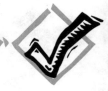

CODE QUESTIONS, NOT ANSWERS

AMOUNT AND CATEGORY SHEET

Directions: This playing board may be made into an overhead transparency.

Air In and Out	Have a Heart	Zap!	Write On	Ready, Set, Go
1	1	1	1	1
2	2	2	2	2
3	3	3	3	3
4	4	4	4	4
5	5	5	5	5

CODE QUESTIONS, NOT ANSWERS

ANSWERS

Directions: This playing board may be made into an overhead transparency.

Air In and Out	Have a Heart	Zap!	Write On	Ready, Set, Go
In Drawer 5 in a large plastic bag	This is the reason that a backboard is kept on the posterior aspect of the code cart	The control the defibrillator must be set on for a "quick look"	The forms distribution center	Establish breathlessness and pulselessness
Needed to intubate a patient but *not* included in Drawer 5	These cause the blood to circulate through the body when performing CPR	Usually the setting to use for the first defibrillation attempt	To the Quality Assessment Department	The two numbers to call to get help on the hospital campus
One of these two people is usually the team leader in a code	What CPR stands for	The maximum amount of energy that can be delivered to a patient from the defibrillator	The reason why the Team Leader must sign the Resuscitation Record	The suction pump is in this drawer
This is what is assessed to verify that the endotracheal tube is in the right place	The place where a pulse check is performed on an adult	"Clear"	The recorder	Use McGill forceps for this
This is used to ventilate the patient before the code cart arrives	The ratio of chest compressions to ventilations in 2-rescuer CPR	This is done to transfer the selected energy into the paddles of the defibrillator	The nurse leader	It is used to do an emergency tracheostomy

CODE QUESTIONS, NOT ANSWERS

QUESTIONS ANSWER KEY

Directions: This playing board may be made into an overhead transparency.

Air In and Out	Have a Heart	Zap!	Write On	Ready, Set, Go
Where is the respiratory equipment?	What provides a hard surface for external chest compressions?	What is "Paddles"?	Where are the resuscitation records available?	What should you do before starting CPR?
What are the laryngoscope handle and blades used for?	What are external chest compressions?	What is 200 joules?	Where does the copy of the resuscitation record get sent?	What are 4444 and 911?
Who is the anesthesiologist or the cardiology resident?	What is cardiopulmonary resuscitation?	What is 360 joules?	What allows the resuscitation record to serve as an order for what is done in a code?	What is in Drawer 4?
What are bilateral breath sounds?	What is the carotid pulse?	What is said before defibrillating a patient?	Who documents the events of a code?	What guides the endotracheal tube down the back of a patient's throat?
What is the mask on the back of the door in the patient's room used for?	What is 5 compressions to 1 breath?	What is "Charge"?	Who runs the cart?	What is the catheterization tray for?

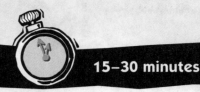

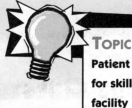

TOOL BOX
Playing boards, lists of rights, small prizes, pens or pencils

BILL OF RIGHTS BINGO

Preparation

1. Calculate how many participants and how many teams of two to six participants you will have.
2. Make a copy of the playing board for each participant.
3. Make one copy of the items sheet for each team and one copy for the educator.
4. Cut one copy of the items sheet between statements so you can mix them for the bingo item callout.
5. Make sure each participant has a pen or pencil.

Implementation

1. Divide the group into two or more teams of two to six learners.
2. Give the group five minutes to list the patient rights in the Bill of Rights.
3. Present the items sheet to each team.
4. Have the learners use the sheet to design their own bingo or Bill of Rights card.
5. The items at the top of the sheet must be included on all their cards. The rest of the squares are filled in from the list at the bottom of the sheet.
6. After completing the cards, play bingo.
7. Award small prizes to the winners.

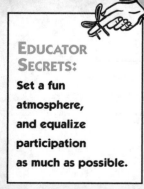

EDUCATOR SECRETS:
Set a fun atmosphere, and equalize participation as much as possible.

By: Amanda Martin, MEd, BSN, RN, CNOR

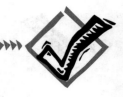

BILL OF RIGHTS BINGO

PLAYING BOARD

This playing board should be copied for each participant.

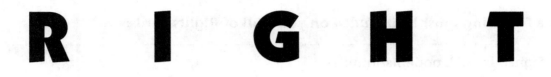

BILL OF RIGHTS BINGO

ITEMS SHEET

Directions: Give one copy to each team. Cut up one copy, and use pieces as callout slips for bingo.

The following must be included on your Bill of Rights cards:

Signed by ALL patients/families
Posted on the unit
Part of the permanent record
All patients must be informed of their rights
All staff should know the rights of the patients
Rights of patients should be respected by caregivers
Nurses are often defenders of patient rights
Rights include personal, health, and legal categories
Patient rights should not be violated

The following may be included on your card. Choose the ones you want, and write one right per square on your card.

Equal consideration for all
Communicate privately with persons of choice
Participate in religious activities of his or her choice
Best possible health care
Confidentiality of medical records
Information about charges for available treatment

continued

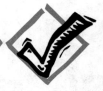

BILL OF RIGHTS BINGO *continued*

Married patients may share a room

Recommend changes without fear of reprisal

Wear personal clothing

Informed consent before participating in experimental research

Equal, appropriate treatment regardless of age, race, color, etc.

Information about available services

Grievances without fear of reprisal, coercion, or discrimination

Adequate notice of transfer or discharge

Grievance mechanisms are in place

Refuse treatment

Freedom from physical/chemical restraints except when authorized by MD

Privacy during care

Retain personal clothing and mementos

Not required to perform services not a part of his or her care plan

Receive personal mail (unopened)

Participate in social activities of his or her choice

Courteous consideration of all

Associate privately with persons of choice

Privacy for visits with spouse

Information regarding medical condition

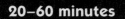
BEWARE: BLOOD BORNE PATHOGENS!

Preparation

1. Determine how many learners will be at your session.

2. Write down some pertinent assignments for your learners
   to do to increase their knowledge about the topic. For example,
   they could demonstrate how they would care for a vial of blood
   that has dropped on the floor and broken or illustrate three ways
   in which blood borne pathogens are spread. You will need two or
   three assignments per team of four to five learners.

3. Gather necessary supplies, personal protective equipment, colored
   pens, drawing board or paper that you might need to demonstrate
   or clarify points to the group.

Implementation

1. Divide the group into teams of four to five.

2. Pick a team leader who can direct and delegate any job
   necessary, so that the team will finish its task in a timely fashion.

3. Let each team randomly pick two to three assignments.

4. Give each team ten minutes to complete the assignment. Then
   have the teams report to the group.

5. Stress or clarify any important points as needed after each team
   has spoken.

By: Mary Arnone Cahoon,
BS, RN

FIRE BRIGADE

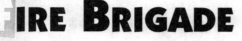

TOOL BOX

Firefighter hats, commissioner badges, dispatcher name tags, evaluator ties, handouts, skit prop box and props, crossword puzzles, answer keys, pens or pencils

Preparation

1. Review the Fire Brigade ready-to-use answer keys to make sure that the information listed agrees with the policies and procedures of your institution. If not, edit them (and the corresponding worksheets) to fit your needs.

2. Determine how many apparel props you need by the number of participants you have. Divide the group into two teams. Each team will then be divided into four work groups.

3. Copy the following ready-to-use sheets, one per participant in each work group: Commissioner A and B worksheets, task sheet, Evaluator worksheet, and Evaluator Reports from the Safety & Security Department. Make a copy of the crossword puzzle for everyone.

4. Copy all the answer sheets for your reference.

5. Collect the prop box contents listed below:

1 coffee pot with flames	1 smoke alarm
1 emergency pull cord	1 manual pull station
1 fire panel	1 telephone
1 gown or pillowcase for smothering the fire	1 CO_2 extinguisher
regular flames (paper)	1 H_2O extinguisher
2 water pitchers	large syringe
poster paper	markers
scissors	tape

6. Make or purchase for each participant in the two teams one of the following: commissioner badges, dispatcher name tags, firefighter hats, and evaluator ties.

7. Make sure each participant has a pen or pencil.

continued

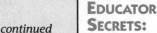

EDUCATOR SECRETS:

Mix the teams so that some experienced people are grouped with newer personnel.

By: Linnea H. Frey, MS, RN
Amanda Martin, MEd, BSN, RN, CNOR

FIRE BRIGADE *continued*

Implementation

1. Divide the participants into teams A and B.

2. Within each team, count off by four.

3. Group 1 is the commissioners; Group 2, the dispatchers; Group 3, the firefighters; and Group 4, the evaluators for teams A and B.

4. After dividing the teams into groups, identify them by name (commissioners, dispatchers, firefighters, or evaluators).

5. Move Team A to one side of the room and Team B to the other side. The evaluators will be at the front of the room; the commissioners, in the next two rows; the dispatchers behind them; and the firefighters in the back.

6. Distribute the badges, name tags, hats, and ties to set the mood.

7. Appoint group leaders. They will take the completed information from one group to the next to facilitate the transition.

8. Distribute the crossword puzzles to all participants. Explain that they should do the puzzles after they have finished or while waiting to begin their tasks.

The First 7 minutes:

9. Give the commissioners the Commissioner A and B worksheets, so that they can read the scenario and come up with the proper steps of response. Be available to answer questions.

10. Give the evaluators the Evaluator A and B task sheet, the Evaluator A and B Worksheet, and the Evaluator Reports. They are to read the reports and use them for cues to fill in the steps on their worksheets. One instructor should help them understand their task by working through the first report synopsis with them and showing them where to place steps on their worksheets. (Allow fifteen to twenty minutes for this activity.)

continued

FIRE BRIGADE *continued*

The Second 7 minutes:

11. Give the dispatchers their task sheet. Their group leader explains the scenario and the steps for response. The dispatchers make sure the steps developed by the commissioners are correct and in the right sequence. If the dispatchers do not agree with the commissioners, the dispatchers make corrections. Then they choose the necessary props and make any others the firefighters will need. They also hold props if necessary.

The Third 7 minutes:

12. When the dispatchers are finished, their leader explains the scenario to the firefighters.

13. The dispatchers who will hold props and the firefighters practice the scenario in the back of the room.

The Fourth 7 minutes:

14. The firefighters from Team A present the scenario to the entire group of learners.

15. The Team A evaluators observe the scenario and, using their evaluation forms, document those items that the firefighters responded to correctly.

16. The Team A dispatchers and commissioners observe the firefighters' response to the mock fires.

17. Repeat Steps 14 through 16 with Team B.

The Last 7 minutes:

18. Evaluators read aloud their evaluation form. All participants agree or disagree with each point on the evaluation form.

19. The educator elaborates on any steps that have been omitted.

The Remaining 10 minutes:

20. This time is to be factored into the introduction, group forming, and details in the forty-five-minute period.

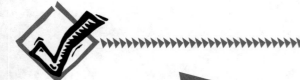

FIRE BRIGADE

COMMISSIONER A: WORKSHEET

Your group has seven minutes to complete its task.

You are charting in the hall. You are told by two visitors that a trash can is on fire in their father's bathroom in room 1377.
How do you respond?
- Complete the following list of steps so that the dispatchers can work on it.
- Complete the crossword puzzle if you have additional time.

Proceed to room 1377.

_____

_____

_____

Pull _____

_____

_____

Hang up the phone.

_____

Direct someone to _____

_____

_____

Extinguish the fire with the _____

_____

FIRE BRIGADE

COMMISSIONER A: WORKSHEET ANSWER KEY

Proceed to room 1377.

Attempt to contain the fire.

Rescue the patient by moving him out of the room.

Close the door to the room.

Pull the manual pull station at the end of the wing.

Call the emergency number.

Tell the operator your name, location, and extension number.

Hang up the phone.

Operator calls back for type, extent of fire, and fire location.

Direct someone to close all doors on unit.

Obtain water extinguisher.

Feel the door before entering with the back of the hand.

Extinguish the fire with the water extinguisher.

Locate the O_2 valve at the request of the Fire Brigade.

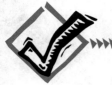

FIRE BRIGADE

COMMISSIONER B: WORKSHEET

Your group has seven minutes to complete its task.

The fire panel on the 14th floor nursing station indicates that a smoke detector on that floor has been activated. You hear the fire chimes sounding. **How do you respond?**
- Complete the following list of steps so that the dispatchers can work on it.
- Complete the crossword puzzle if you have additional time.

Proceed to the fire panel.

_____

Push _____

_____

A flaming coffee pot is found in the kitchen.

_____

_____

Direct someone to _____

_____

_____

_____

_____

_____

Extinguish the fire with the _____

_____

Locate the O_2 control valve at the request of the Fire Brigade.

Copyright © 1995 by Mosby–Year Book, Inc.

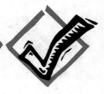

FIRE BRIGADE

COMMISSIONER B: WORKSHEET ANSWER KEY

Proceed to the fire panel.

Note area where fire detector has been activated.

Push button to acknowledge first-stage alarm.

Investigate the area designated for fire.

A flaming coffee pot is found in the kitchen.

Unplug the coffee pot, attempt to contain the fire.

Close the door to the room.

Direct someone to dial the emergency number if the operator

hasn't called you.

Tell the operator your name, unit location, and extension number

and then hang up.

The operator calls back for type, extent of fire, and room number.

Direct someone to close all doors on unit.

Locate the CO_2 extinguisher.

Extinguish the fire with the CO_2 extinguisher.

Expect response from Fire Brigade.

Locate the O_2 control valve at the request of the Fire Brigade.

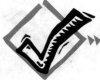

Fire Brigade

Task Sheets

Give a copy of these instructions to each group.

Dispatcher A and B Task Sheet:

Your group has seven minutes to complete the following tasks:
- Take the scenario from the commissioner's group and make sure the steps are correct and in the right sequence.
- Make changes as needed.
- Pick how many characters you need in the scenario that will be acted out by the firefighters. Dispatchers may assist the firefighters by holding props during the performance.
- Pick out the props from the prop box that the firefighters need to act out the scenario.
- Make any other needed props.
- One member of your group explains the scenario and props to the firefighters. You must ensure that the firefighters can act out the scenario step by step with the appropriate props.
- Complete the crossword puzzle if you have additional time.

Firefighter A and B Task Sheet:

Your group has seven minutes to complete the following tasks:
- Take the scenario from the dispatchers.
- Decide who will act in the scenario.
- Get the props for the scenario from the dispatchers.
- Act out the scenario step by step with the appropriate props. Dispatchers may aid in holding props.
- Complete the crossword puzzle if you have additional time.

FIRE BRIGADE

TASK SHEETS *continued*

Evaluator A and B Task Sheet:

Your group has fifteen to twenty minutes to complete the following tasks:

- Look at the evaluation form given to you to evaluate the scenarios that the firefighters will enact.
- Read the Evaluator Reports of fire drills from the Safety & Security Department.
- Identify mistakes made as indicated from the reports.
- Discuss the proper response to each mistake.
- List these proper responses on your evaluation report where appropriate.
- Are there any steps missing from the evaluation form? If so, fill them in.
- Watch your group's scenario.
- Grade the scenario step by step with the items on your evaluation form (and those filled in by your group) to see if the proper response was made.
- Complete the crossword puzzle if you have additional time.

FIRE BRIGADE

EVALUATOR A AND B WORKSHEET

Evaluation

Rescue

Were persons in immediate danger moved to safety? _____

Were electrical safety measures used? _____

Alarm

Which manual pull station was activated? _____

_____ _____

_____ _____

_____ _____

_____ _____

Confine

Were all room doors closed? _____

_____ _____

Extinguish

Were materials available to smother the fire? _____

_____ _____

_____ _____

_____ _____

Fire Brigade

Evaluator A and B Worksheet Answer Key

Evaluation

Rescue

Were persons in immediate danger moved to safety? _____

Were electrical safety measures used? _____

Alarm

Which manual pull station was activated? _____

Was the emergency number utilized? _____

Did the person hang up so that the operator could call back? _____

Did the person check the fire panel? _____

Did the personnel respond to the chime alarm? _____

Confine

Were all room doors closed? _____

Were any patients in the room moved away from the fire? _____

Extinguish

Were materials available to smother the fire? _____

Was the proper extinguisher used? _____

Did the person aim at the base of the fire? _____

Did they test the door with the back of the hand before entering? _____

FIRE BRIGADE

EVALUATOR REPORTS FROM THE SAFETY & SECURITY DEPARTMENT

Report #1: The fire drill was conducted on the 15th floor of the hospital. An electrical fire was simulated by placing a red flag on electrical equipment in the room adjacent to the nursing station. A red card was given to Nurse F. Ire. Nurse Ire proceeded to the affected area and directed Nurse Jones to call the operator or "0" and indicate that a Code Red was on the 15th floor. The rest of the drill was handled well.

Report #2: A simulated electrical fire was activated on the 15th floor of the hospital in the utility room. A notification card was given to S. Smith who said she did not know how to respond. She asked other employees for help and did not receive it. Finally, after six minutes another nurse went through the RACE procedure. The manual pull station location was not immediately known, and when finally directed to it, Nurse Smith punched it. An unknown employee yelled, "Fire!" and alarmed the patients.

Report #3: In September, a simulated electrical fire was activated in the south wing of the 15th floor. A red card was given to B. Boop. Nurse Boop went to the room, looked at the fire, and ran to the nurses' station to tell her fellow workers. The other nurses began closing doors to rooms while Nurse Boop called the operator dialing the emergency number. She ran back to the hall and then closed the door to the affected room. The affected room and the nurses' station are at opposite ends of the hall. None of the nurses pulled the manual pull station, nor did they get a fire extinguisher.

Report #4: In May, a red card was given to Nurse F. Browning. She checked the room to confirm a trash fire and proceeded to advise the control desk personnel of the situation. She returned to the west wing and closed the door to several of the rooms on the wing, except the door across the hall from the fire. F. Browning returned to the room with a water extinguisher to simulate putting out the fire, and the rest of the drill proceeded correctly.

Report #5: Nurse Dial performed well during the drill. She delegated responsibility well to other nurses so that she could keep her attention on the fire. When she returned to the closed door with the fire extinguisher, she immediately entered the room.

Report #6: A doll was placed in room 1530 to simulate a child playing with matches. A red card given to Nurse K. Close said that there was a trash can fire in room 1530. She proceeded to the room and closed the door. She did not remove the doll from the room. She obtained a CO_2 extinguisher and pretended to douse the flames.

Report #7: A fire drill notice card was given to Nurse N. Moe. Ms. Moe was also told that there was a simulated trash can fire in the solarium. The notice card said that the can and nearby chairs had also caught on fire. Ms. Moe said she was too busy to participate in the drill. She then changed her mind and participated. She pulled the manual pull station by the solarium. She then dialed the correct emergency number. After searching for the correct extinguisher, she was unable to locate it. Nurse Moe said, "The writing on the door said, 'fire hose,' so that's what I thought it was, not an extinguisher."

Report #8: A smoke detector was activated on the 15th floor. No action was taken.

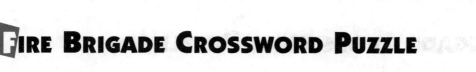

FIRE BRIGADE CROSSWORD PUZZLE

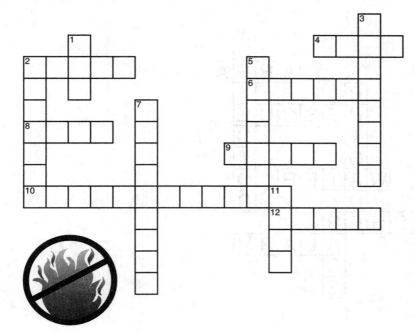

Across

2. When there is a fire, we do this to all doors
4. A smoke detector allows you to know which _____ the fire is in
6. This is the first step in the RACE process
8. We aim at the base of this with an extinguisher
9. We use this type of extinguisher for a paper fire
10. CO$_2$ and water are two kinds of this
12. We must call this in when there is a fire

Down

1. This extinguisher is used for electrical fires
2. This is the 3rd step in the RACE process
3. This allows us to know where the fire is in the early stages
5. This team responds to all fire alarms
7. We want to notify this operator
11. This is the acronym that helps us remember the process to follow in a fire emergency

Fire Brigade Crossword Puzzle

Answer Key

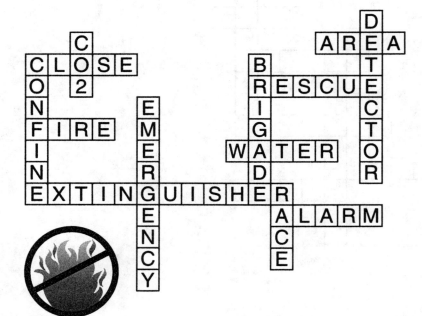

Across

2. close
4. area
6. rescue
8. fire
9. water
10. extinguisher
12. alarm

Down

1. CO$_2$
2. confine
3. detector
5. brigade
7. emergency
11. RACE

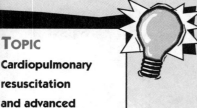

TOOL BOX
Codeword crossword puzzle, pens or pencils, answer key

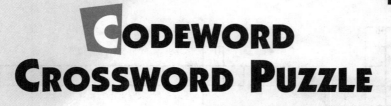

CODEWORD CROSSWORD PUZZLE

Preparation

1. Make a copy of the ready-to-use Codeword crossword puzzle for each participant.
2. Use this as an introduction to the lesson or as a review after the lesson.
3. Make sure each participant has a pen or pencil.
4. Make a copy of the answer key.

Variation

1. Use a poster printer copy machine to turn the crossword into a poster-size image.
2. Plan for groups of two to six to discuss and fill in a poster-size copy of the crossword puzzle before or after your lesson.

Implementation

1. Pass out the large or small crossword puzzle.
2. Challenge your learners to complete the puzzle as individuals or as teams.
3. If energy and attention are low during your lesson presentation, stop and let your participants engage in this energizing activity.
4. Crossword puzzles can also be sent out days or weeks after the lesson as reinforcement of important concepts.

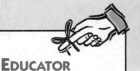

EDUCATOR SECRETS:
If you have different ability levels in your session, pair learners to maximize benefits to all.

By: Michele Deck, MEd, BSN, RN, ACCE-R
Jeanne Silva, BSN, RN, CCRN

CODEWORD CROSSWORD PUZZLE

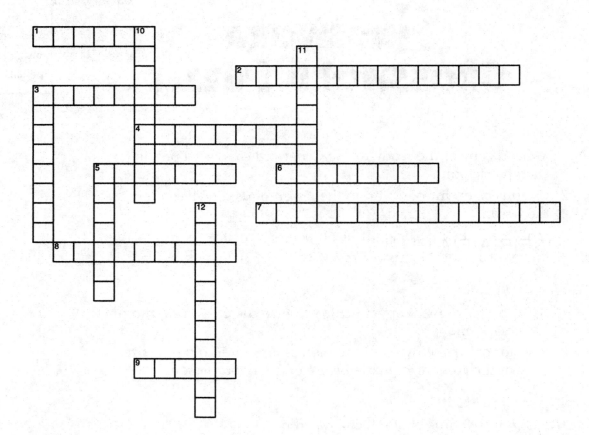

Supine

1. Reverses metabolic acidosis
2. For treatment of anaphylactic shock/septic shock
3. For treatment of arrhythmias due to digitalis toxicity
4. For treatment of ventricular tach; decreased conduction velocity/calms the heart down
5. For treatment of bradyarrhythmias; given only IV
6. Cardiac vagolytic, decreases input from the vagus nerve
7. For treatment of EMD pattern on monitor, but patient has no pulse
8. For supraventricular tachycardia, blocks rapid ineffective conduction
9. For treatment of pulmonary edema or increased intercranial pressure

Erect

3. Used for elevation of blood pressure
5. A noncardioselective beta blocker
10. For early use in V-fib, for V-tach when Lidocaine and Pronestyl are ineffective
11. Decreased conduction velocity; for treatment of V-tach used if Lidocaine ineffective or allergic
12. Increased myocardial contractile force; cardiac stimulant

Codeword Crossword Puzzle

Answer Key

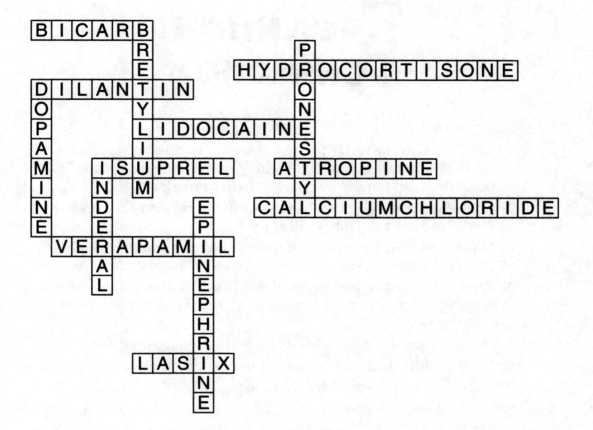

Supine

1. bicarb
2. hydrocortisone
3. Dilantin
4. lidocaine
5. Isuprel
6. atropine
7. calcium chloride
8. Verapamil
9. Lasix

Erect

3. dopamine
5. Inderal
10. bretylium
11. Pronestyl
12. epinephrine

HOW DID YOU DO?

11–12 Participate in ALL codes in your area.
8–10 Start your drug cards NOW.
6–9 Check the code cart DAILY.
1–5 Attend ALL sessions of Code review.

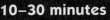
TOPIC
Common causes
of nosocomial
infections and
work-related injuries

TOOL BOX
Bugman and
Prevention Gretchen
panel signs,
prevention
connection game
board, emcee
question cards,
panel answer cards

PREVENTION CONNECTION

Preparation

1. Read through the ready-to-use Prevention Connection game questions. If they do not agree with your institution's policies, procedures, and information, edit them as needed.

2. Copy each game question, correct answer, and distractor on a 3" x 5" index card. This is called set A.

3. Make a second identical set of these cards, and call it set B. One set is for your use; one set is for the panel members to read.

4. On a poster board, glue eighteen envelopes so that they are open. Number them from one to eighteen on the side of the envelope that shows.

5. Place one index card in each of the envelopes from set A.

6. Place the identical card from set B in the envelopes.

7. Copy the ready-to-use panel sign pages.

8. Cut the signs apart on the dotted lines, so that you have nine Prevention Gretchens and nine Bugman signs.

9. Place three chairs side by side in the front of the room for the emcee and the contestants.

10. Place chairs in three rows of three in the front of the room for the panel.

11. Place the poster in front of the room where it can be easily seen.

12. Recruit willing participants at the start of the session.

continued

EDUCATOR SECRETS:
Divide the room into two teams and have one side cheer for each contestant.

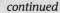
By: Rosalie Barker, BSN, RNC
Bonnie Maestri, MN, RNC, ACCE

PREVENTION CONNECTION *continued*

Implementation

1. As the educator, you will act as the emcee.

2. Ask for eleven volunteers. Two will act as contestants; nine, as panel members. Describe the game rules to everyone.

3. The two contestants will be identified as "Bugman" and "Gretchen."

4. The emcee will toss a coin to see who goes first.

5. The first contestant will pick a panel member.

6. The emcee will turn to the envelope poster board and pick a question card. Prior to reading the question, the emcee hands a duplicate question card that contains the correct answer and a distractor response to the designated panel member.

7. The panel member has the option of responding to the question read aloud by the emcee with either the correct answer or the distractor.

8. The emcee asks the contestant if he or she agrees or disagrees and allows time for him or her to consult with the rest of the panel.

9. If the contestant agrees or disagrees as appropriate, he or she wins the square and the panel member holds up his or her sign with "Bugman" or "Gretchen."

10. The first contestant to achieve three in a row wins the games. More than one game can be played to cover all the concepts.

PREVENTION CONNECTION

GAME QUESTIONS

Directions: Place one question/answer on a 3" x 5" index card. Make 2 identical sets. Mark the back of each card in one set with an "A" and the other set with a "B."

1. What is Stickgard?

Correct Answer: *A safety needle product designed to prevent accidental needle stick injuries*

Distractor: *A deodorant for trees*

2. Where can Stickgard safety needles be found?

Correct Answer: *They are located on the nonchargeable supply cart.*

Distractor: *On the shores of Lake Ponchartrain*

3. How often should a central line dressing change occur?

Correct Answer: *Every seven days or prn if necessary*

Distractor: *Every three days*

4. How often should a central line site be assessed?

Correct Answer: *At least once a shift*

Distractor: *Every twenty-four hours*

5. What are the signs and symptoms of central line infection?

Correct Answer: *Redness, swelling, fever, increased WBCs, drainage*

Distractor: *Shivering, trembling, and loss of bladder control*

6. What does nosocomial infection mean?

Correct Answer: *An infection that occurs during or after hospitalization and that was neither present nor incubating at the time of admission*

Distractor: *An infection that occurs when not practicing safe sex*

7. What are Universal Precautions?

Correct Answer: *Safety measures used by all employees to prevent disease transmission through blood or body fluids exposure*

Distractor: *Strategies developed by the Pentagon to protect the world from Saddam Hussein*

8. What is the most important means for prevention of nosocomial infections?

Correct Answer: *Good handwashing before and after contact with every patient*

Distractor: *Refuse the patient admission to the hospital*

9. True or false: All health care personnel are responsible for decreasing the incidence of nosocomial infections.

Correct Answer: *True*

Distractor: *False*

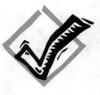

PREVENTION CONNECTION

10. When should you use a Stickgard safety needle?

Correct Answer: *When administering IVPB and IVP drugs and when drawing blood from a central line*

Distractor: *When mending a button on a resident's lab coat*

11. True or false: Stickgard comes with an 18-gauge needle only.

Correct Answer: *False*

Distractor: *True*

12. True or false: Documentation of central line dressing change is not necessary as long as the procedure is done.

Correct Answer: *False*

Distractor: *True*

13. How often should you change the Stickgard safety needle?

Correct Answer: *It is a single-use item and should be discarded after each drug administration.*

Distractor: *Every seventy-two hours with IV tubing change*

14. What preparation should be used before entering a central line port?

Correct Answer: *Betadine, let dry for one minute, then alcohol*

Distractor: *Preparation H*

15. What is the most common mode of transmission for nosocomial infection?

Correct Answer: *Direct contact*

Distractor: *Poor sterile technique*

16. What are the most common measures used when practicing Universal Precautions?

Correct Answer: *Good handwashing, gloves, sharps containers, and gown, mask, and goggles when appropriate*

Distractor: *Abstinence or the use of condoms and diaphragms*

17. Besides handwashing, name another method to prevent the spread of infection.

Correct Answer: *Identify patients at risk and properly dispose of trash and waste.*

Distractor: *Destroy all "dead wood" on your unit.*

18. True or false: When health care workers are potentially exposed to Hepatitis B or HIV, they should first fill out the employee accident report form and then notify their supervisor.

Correct Answer: *False. The employee should immediately cleanse the area and then report to employee health.*

Distractor: *True*

PREVENTION **C**ONNECTION

PANEL **SIGNS**

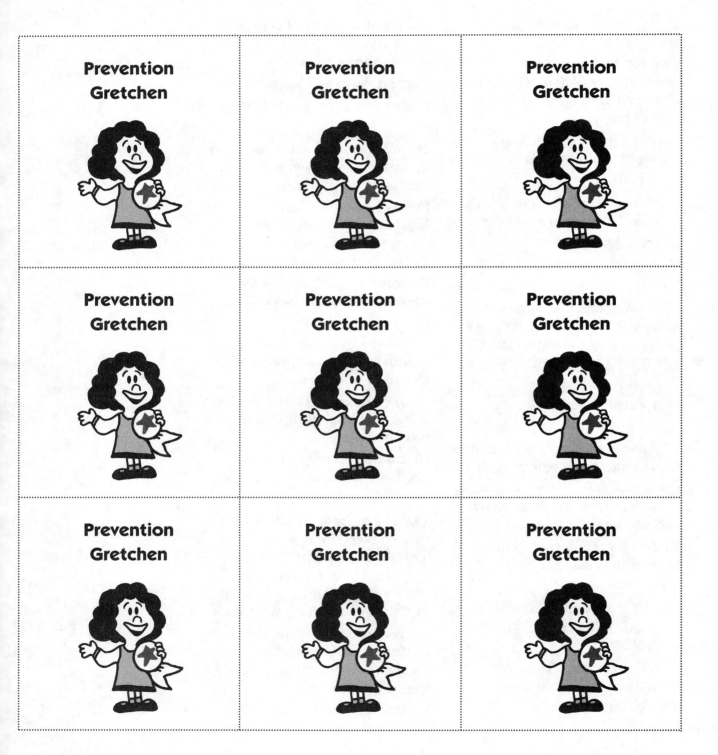

PREVENTION **C**ONNECTION

PANEL **SIGNS** *continued*

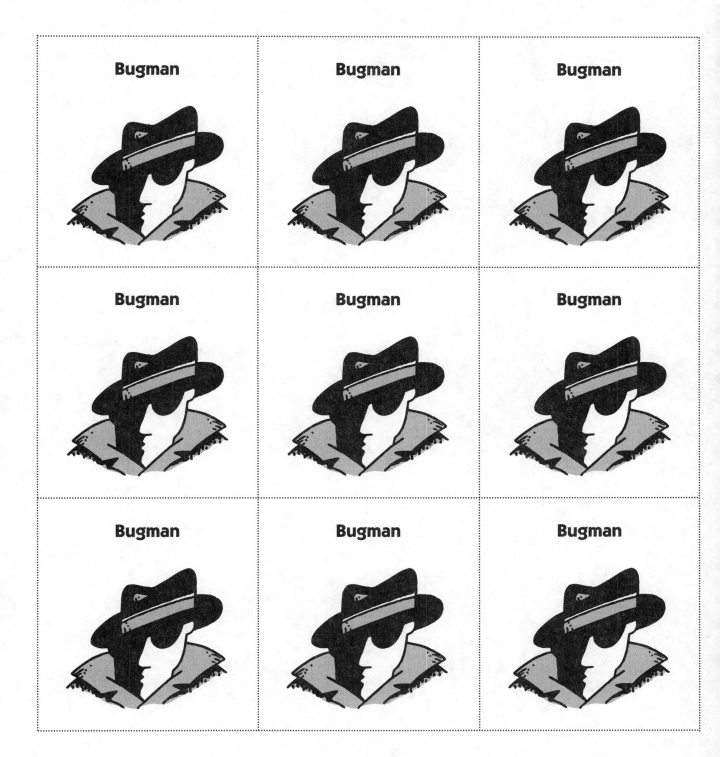

87

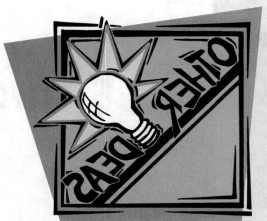

PART 3

INSTANT TOOLS FOR LEARNING IDEAS

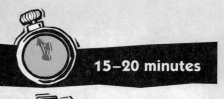

15–20 minutes

TOOL BOX
Bingo sheets,
pens or pencils,
small prize

TOPIC
Networking tool to
help participants
meet and remember
each other

PEOPLE BINGO

Preparation

1. Make enough copies of the bingo sheet for all the participants and for the instructor.
2. Distribute the copies.
3. Make sure each participant has a pen or pencil.

Implementation

1. Invite the participants to mingle, obtaining a signature in each square of the bingo sheet.
2. To obtain signatures, they must ask questions, using the bingo sheets for prompts. For example, "Have you worked here ten years or more?" or "Do you love dogs?" The participants cannot hand it to someone and say, "Just fill in your name where it fits."
3. The object is to have a signature in each box. If your group is smaller than twenty-one, participants may sign up to three boxes per sheet.
4. Then play bingo with the signed sheets. Using your copy of the bingo sheet, call out the information from one of the boxes.
5. Ask participants to X out the box on their sheet if it is signed. If it is not signed, they are not to mark it off.
6. Continue calling out box information until someone gets bingo horizontally, vertically, or diagonally. That person receives a small prize.

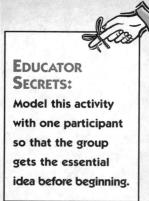

EDUCATOR SECRETS:
Model this activity
with one participant
so that the group
gets the essential
idea before beginning.

By: Nancy Hennen, BSN, RNC

PEOPLE BINGO

Worked here ten years or more	Has brown eyes	Plays a musical instrument	Comes from a large family
Loves dogs	Works in the same area as you	Speaks a foreign language	Born to shop
Worked New Year's last year	Has seen the Flintstones	Was born at this hospital	Works on third floor
Works on sixth floor	Has a "green thumb"	Has worked at our facility less than two years	Has a five-year anniversary working here
Takes a trip every year	Has been to the employee Christmas party	Went to a fundraiser	Works D/E shift

TOOL BOX
Colored plastic eggs,
small gift-wrapped
boxes or balloons,
tips typed on strips
of paper, small
goodies for prizes

TIPS TREASURE HUNT

Preparation

1. Create tips or ideas on subject matter you are teaching.
2. Print or type tips or ideas on a sheet of paper.
3. Cut the sheets so that each tip or idea is on a small separate piece of paper.
4. Obtain some plastic eggs, gift boxes, or balloons.
5. Place one tip or idea in each egg, box, or balloon. If using boxes, wrap them. If using balloons, inflate them.
6. Place the items around the room during a break.
7. Divide group into teams.

Implementation

1. Participants are offered a number of tips or ideas on how to perform the different professional roles they assume.
2. When the participants return from a break, direct them to find the hidden eggs or gift boxes.
3. Ask them to open these and read the tips aloud.
4. If using balloons, hand out balloons to each team. Ask participants to pop the balloons without using a sharp object.
5. Award points to the teams for the tips found by their members.
6. Points acquired during the program are exchanged at the end for a goody!

EDUCATOR
SECRETS:
Popping balloons
are noisy, so choose
your meeting room
carefully.

By: Sherry Haizlip, BSN, RN, C

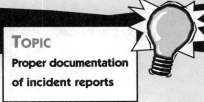
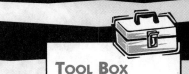

TOOL BOX
Instructions,
character dossiers,
incomplete story
line, incident report
forms for your facility,
pens or pencils

How to Host an Incident Investigation

Preparation

1. Copy enough ready-to-use character dossiers so that each participant has one.
2. Copy enough ready-to-use incomplete story lines so that each group of twelve participants has one.
3. Obtain copies of your facility's incident report form, one per participant.
4. Make sure each participant has a pen or pencil.

Implementation

1. Divide participants into groups of twelve players.
2. Distribute the character dossiers.
3. Allow each person to choose a character to portray.
4. Distribute a copy of the incomplete story line to each group.
5. Distribute incident report forms.
6. Each group has twenty minutes to complete the story line and the incident report and to list the ways the incident could have been avoided.
7. Compare and discuss findings together. Everyone wins because their knowledge of accident/incident prevention has increased.

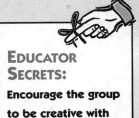

EDUCATOR SECRETS:
Encourage the group to be creative with the activity.

By: Tina Johnson, BS

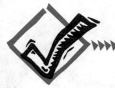

How to Host an Incident Investigation

Incomplete Story Line

Main Event at the Shady Rest Center

The Shady Rest is a seventy-bed center filled to capacity 360 days a year. The center is located on a tree-lined road that winds through the valley surrounding the Great Smoky Mountains in North Carolina. The Shady Rest Center is situated on approximately twenty acres of beautifully manicured grounds.

It is a cool summer evening in 1995, and the lives of the staff and residents at the Shady Rest Center are about to change dramatically. The events of this ill-fated night unfold as follows:

It is Tuesday. Around 9:15 pm, Mrs. Oldhappy turns on her call light to summon help. CNA Candy Dropher responds to the light. On her way, Candy slips and falls in a puddle of urine on the floor. As Candy rises to her feet, she feels a slight pop in her back.

By this time Mrs. Oldhappy is yelling, "Someone come help me. I've been waiting a long time!" Candy knows that since Mrs. Oldhappy broke her arm, she has needed special attention with her cast. Before the CNA can ask what is wrong, Mrs. Oldhappy hits Candy on the side of the head with the cast.

CNA Pam Handler sees Candy fall onto the floor and, of course, hears Mrs. Oldhappy yelling for help. The call light is still on, so Pam goes to see if she can help Candy and Mrs. Oldhappy. As Pam enters Mrs. Oldhappy's room, she finds Candy unconscious on the floor. Pam bends down to check on Candy, making Mrs. Oldhappy very angry. Pam continues to check on Candy, and Mrs. Oldhappy bends down and bites Pam on the arm.

Pam becomes irritated and leaves the room to get help from the DON, Ivy Therapy, and the ADON, Jon Helpsalot. By the time they return to the room, Mrs. Oldhappy is hysterical. Ivy approaches Mrs. Oldhappy and attempts to calm her down while Jon and Pam take care of Candy.

How to Host an Incident Investigation

Character Dossier

The cast of Shady characters:

You are Mrs. Helen Oldhappy, and you are a resident at the Shady Rest Center. The following are facts pertaining to your stay at the Shady Rest Center:

- You are seventy-five years old.
- You do not have a history of combative behavior.
- You have not shown previous signs of confusion.
- You are usually very happy and a pleasure to have as a resident.

You are Ms. Candy Dropher, a CNA for the Shady Rest Center. The following are facts you should know:

- You work the evening shift at the Shady Rest Center.
- Your shift has been one person short due to an illness.
- You have been working at the Shady Rest Center for five years.

You are Ms. Pam Handler, a CNA for the Shady Rest Center. The following information regarding your employment is pertinent:

- You work full-time on the night shift.
- You volunteered to work double shifts to cover for the short evening shift.
- You have been employed with the Shady Rest Center for five years.

You are Ms. Ivy Therapy, the DON at the Shady Rest Center. The following are pertinent facts regarding your employment:

- You work full-time as DON for the Shady Rest Center.
- You have been employed in the capacity of DON for fifteen years.
- Your normal shift is days.

continued

95

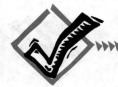

How to Host an
Incident Investigation *continued*

Character Dossier

You are Mr. Jon Helpsalot, the ADON for the Shady Rest Center. The following is information regarding your employment at the Shady Rest Center:
- You are a full-time RN working the evening shift at the Shady Rest Center.
- You worked for the Shady Rest Center part-time as an LPN while you finished your RN degree.
- As a company benefit, the Shady Rest Center helped pay for your RN degree.

You are Mr. Randy Dropher, the spouse of CNA Candy Dropher. The following facts pertain to your role in the incident:
- You don't like the hours that Candy works at the center. You would like Candy to work the day shift.
- You are contacted by the Shady Rest Center after Candy is injured.

You are Dr. Noah Heart, and you are the medical director for the Shady Rest Center. The following are facts that you should know:
- All incidents are reported to you.
- You must examine all people with injuries or have medical reports transferred to you by the attending physician.
- You have worked with the Shady Rest Center as a medical director for five years.

You are Ms. Penny Pincher, the administrator for the Shady Rest Center. The following are facts that the administrator should know:
- You are responsible for the lives and safety of both residents and employees.
- You are accountable for and must sign all incident reports.
- Resident family members may file grievances against employees, residents, and other family members with the administrator.

continued

How to Host an
Incident Investigation *continued*

Character Dossier

You are Mr. Malcolm Practice, attorney at law. The following are facts that pertain to your role in the incident:
- You are Minnie Practice's son.
- You pay for Mrs. Practice's stay at the center.
- You are a very prominent attorney in Petticoat Junction.
- You work primarily with personal injury cases.

You are Mrs. Minnie Practice, a resident of the Shady Rest Center. The following are facts pertaining to you and your stay at the Shady Rest Center:
- You are Helen Oldhappy's roommate and have been since your admission.
- Your son is a prominent lawyer in Petticoat Junction and you are very proud of him.
- You have a history of being involved in incidents at the center.

You are Ms. Wilma H. Resource, the human resource director for the Shady Rest Center. The center has an active employee base of seventy-six. The following are facts the human resource director should know:
- The most accidents and/or incidents occur on Tuesdays.
- The human resource director is responsible for processing and maintaining records based on accident or incident reports.

You are Ms. Ima Safeplayer, the safety coordinator for the Shady Rest Center. The following are facts the safety coordinator should know:
- Accidents and/or incidents most frequently occur on Tuesdays.
- All incidents must be reported immediately.
- Wet floors should be identified with a wet floor sign.
- It is everyone's job to watch for wet floors and to notify the appropriate people to take care of the situation.
- Employees' on-the-job injuries, both physically and financially, affect everyone—the injured employee, coworkers, and the company.

15–30 minutes

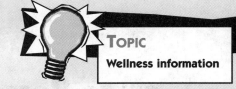
TOOL BOX

Questions, overhead projector, prizes, buzzing device or bell, transparency pen, answer key

WELLNESS SERVICES FAMILY SQUABBLE

Preparation

1. Have the ready-to-use questions made into an overhead transparency.
2. Place the transparency on the bed of the overhead. Mask the overhead transparency with a sheet of paper.
3. Obtain two buzzing devices or bells, one for each team.
4. Have a transparency pen to write answers on the overhead transparency.
5. Make a copy of the answer key.

Implementation

1. Begin a meeting with this activity to warm everyone up and to impart information. The questions are designed with humor as an icebreaker but then lead into knowledge, information, or review about the department or company.
2. Divide your group into two teams of equal number and experience.
3. Introduce and use a buzzing device or bell for each team to ring in.
4. One representative from each team stands by the buzzer or bell.
5. Reveal the first question.
6. The team who buzzes or rings first gets to proceed with the question, provided their first response is correct; otherwise the opposing team gets to proceed.
7. Write in the correct answers on the overhead transparency as they are given (refer to the answer key).
8. One point per correct answer is awarded.
9. The team is allowed three incorrect answers or strikes per question before the other team gets to steal the points accumulated by coming up with another correct answer to the question.
10. Continue until all questions have been answered. Award prizes at the end. Prizes are a new car (child's party favor) for the winning team and a watch (child's party favor) for the second place team.

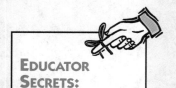

EDUCATOR SECRETS:

Equalize participation as much as possible.

By: Suzi Weigel, MA

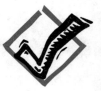

WELLNESS SERVICES FAMILY SQUABBLE

QUESTIONS

Name five relatives of Elvis Presley.

_____   _____

_____   _____

_____

Name six reasons to own a van in Wellness Services.

_____   _____

_____   _____

_____   _____

Name seven components of the Wellness Wheel.

_____   _____

_____   _____

_____   _____

_____

Name the vice presidents of our hospital.

_____   _____

_____   _____

Name the top business contracts with Wellness Services.

_____   _____

_____   _____

Name seven accomplishments achieved by Wellness Services last year.

_____   _____

_____   _____

_____   _____

_____

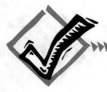

WELLNESS SERVICES FAMILY SQUABBLE

ANSWER KEY

Name five relatives of Elvis Presley.
- Vernon (father)
- Gladys (mother)
- Priscilla (wife)
- Lisa Marie (daughter)
- Jessie Garon (twin brother)

Name six reasons to own a van in Wellness Services.
- Transport equipment to health screenings
- Transport staff to lunch
- Carpool kids
- Take dogs to vet
- Groceries
- Camping

Name seven components of the Wellness Wheel.
- Exercise
- Diet
- Body weight
- Smoking cessation
- Stress management
- Auto safety
- Personal hygiene

Name the vice presidents of our hospital.
- (Fill in own information.)

Name the top business contracts with Wellness Services.
- (Fill in own information.)

Name seven accomplishments achieved by Wellness Services last year.
- (Fill in own information.)

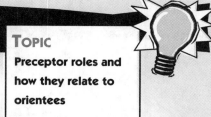

TOPIC
Preceptor roles and
how they relate to
orientees

TOOL BOX
Six 50-piece puzzles,
instructions for
preceptors

PRECEPTOR PUZZLE

Preparation

1. Obtain six 50-piece puzzles.
2. Place each puzzle in a sealable bag.
3. Copy the ready-to-use instructions page.
4. Cut the page along the six lines.
5. Place one set of instructions in each puzzle bag.
6. When you are inserting Instruction 3 into a bag, remove about five pieces of the puzzle and keep them with you.

Implementation

1. Divide the group into six teams.
2. Select a preceptor from each team, and instruct them separately from the rest of the group.
3. Give each preceptor a copy of their assigned scenario.
4. Tell the preceptors the following: "The object of the game is to be the first group to totally complete the puzzle; preceptors' behavior should elicit team responses; preceptors should not deviate from the scenario; the activity is not timed; preceptors should not share their scenario with anyone, not even with their teams."
5. Distribute the puzzles and say, "Go!"
6. After the teams play out their roles, stop the activity and debrief the teams.
7. Have the preceptors read their scenarios.
8. Have each team tell how they feel about their preceptor.
9. Discuss how the preceptors felt.
10. Compare and contrast the positive and negative aspects of behavior.

The six different preceptor instructions follow on the ready-to-use page.

EDUCATOR
SECRETS:

Appoint group
observers to record
responses to the
situations. This
allows for interesting
discussion during
the debrief.

By: Martha Dardenne, BSN, RN
Nancy Hennen, BSN, RNC

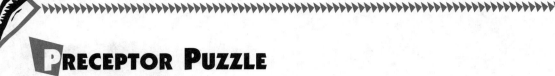

PRECEPTOR PUZZLE

PRECEPTOR INSTRUCTIONS

1. Please return to your group of orientees and complete the puzzle by yourself. Say things like, "I'd rather do it myself," "I don't have time to explain," and "It's too complicated for you to do," "This is so stupid."

2. Please return to your group of orientees and be supportive, motivating, and encouraging. Do and say anything it takes for your group of orientees to succeed.

3. Unfortunately, your group is missing some of the pieces (it's a secret). You may say things like "Nothing ever works around here," "Better get used to this," or "In the good old days, this would have never happened."

4. Say and do very little to guide your group of orientees. Feel free to take a break.

5. Be very competitive. You want to be finished first no matter what. Remember a completed puzzle can look like whatever the group wants. Say things like, "We've got to win," "Got to be the best," or "Got to get this done."

6. Please return to your group of orientees and follow this detailed list of instructions. Tell your orientees: "Don't do anything until I tell you," "Open the plastic bag. Dump the puzzle on the table. Group the pieces by color. Put the inside pieces together first. Put the edge pieces on last." You may also say things like: "This is the way we do it here," "Trust me I know best," and "My way is the only way."

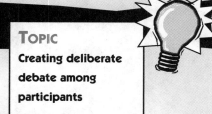

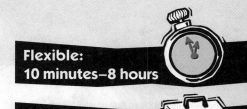

TOOL BOX
Red, yellow, blue,
and green cards,
dots, name tags,
small prize

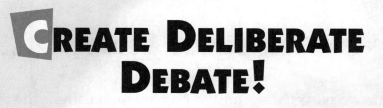

CREATE DELIBERATE DEBATE!

Preparation

1. Obtain red, yellow, blue, and green construction paper.
2. Cut each sheet into four equal parts.
3. Make enough parts so that each participant can have one square of each color.
4. Distribute the squares to participants as they enter or place the squares at each participant's chair.
5. Obtain a pack of multicolored dots.
6. Make sure each participant has a name tag.
7. Make a list of unknown facts, unpopular statements, and/or "sacred cows" that will motivate participants to respond.

Implementation

1. The process of deliberate debate involves the educator presenting unknown facts, unpopular statements, and/or "sacred cows" that motivate participants to respond.
2. Invite participants to respond by choosing a colored piece of paper and waving it in the air:

   Red   "It won't work!"

   Yellow   "Yes, but what about . . . ?"

   Blue   "Moooooo" (a sacred cow means "We've always done it that way!")

   Green   "Okay with me!"

continued

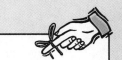

EDUCATOR SECRETS:
Assure that adequate
discussion ensues to
allow learners to deal
with the feelings that
emerge.

By: Linda Brazen, MSN, RN,
C, CNOR

CREATE DELIBERATE DEBATE! *continued*

3. Any time a participant wants to respond to something, he or she immediately picks up the colored card and waves it in the air.

4. As soon as one person starts to wave a card in the air, everyone in the room must pick up the color card that most represents his or her response to what was said and waves it in the air.

5. The educator gives the first person to wave a card a dot.

6. Take a quick survey of the responses by looking at the color of the cards being waved, and entertain any discussion.

7. The learner with the most dots at the end of the session wins a prize.

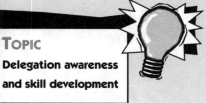
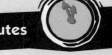

20–30 minutes

BLIND DELEGATION

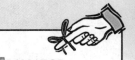

TOOL BOX

Sugar cubes, opaque
bags, blindfolds, flat
surface for building,
flipchart, pens or
pencils

Preparation

1. Place fifteen sugar cubes in an opaque bag and close the top.
2. Make enough bags so that each team of three receives one bag.
3. Copy one set of ready-to-use instructions A and B per team and cut them apart on the lines provided.
4. Distribute one blindfold per team.
5. Copy one ready-to-use question page per team.
6. Set up a flipchart for debriefing at completion of the activity.
7. Make sure each participant has a pen or pencil.

Implementation

1. Introduce this as an exercise in delegation.
2. Divide the participants into threes: one observer, one delegator, and one builder in each group. Give the observers a bag of sugar cubes and their Part A instructions. Give the delegators and builders their Part A instructions. Give all the groups two minutes to read their Part A instructions.
3. Builders place a blindfold or mask over their eyes and follow the instructions given to them. The observers time exercise A.
4. Hand out Part B instructions. Strategy and planning now occur as prompted by these instructions.
5. The observers time exercise B.
6. The questions handout is given to all three team members. The leader places it on the table during the second try.
7. Delegators, builders, and observers share their thoughts in this order.
8. Group draws conclusions about when and how to delegate and lists these on a flipchart page.
9. Each person is asked to write down one idea to take to his or her workplace.

EDUCATOR
SECRETS:

Use an eyeglass
mask for those who
do not wish to be
blindfolded.

BLIND DELEGATION

INSTRUCTIONS PART A

Directions: Copy and cut apart for participants.

Instructions A: Delegator

1. You will have the builder build a tower of singular pieces as high as possible in three minutes. If the tower falls, you must wait thirty seconds before starting again.

2. You may not touch the tower or your builder. You can use verbal instructions only.

3. Do not talk to the builder until the observer starts timing.

Instructions A: Builder

1. You will be given building materials by the observer when the timing begins.

2. The delegator will give you verbal directions only and will not touch you or the building materials.

3. Please put on the blindfold provided by the observer just before the time begins.

4. Use your nondominant hand to build with.

Instructions A: Observer

1. You will give the builder the blindfold and the bag of building materials just prior to timing.

2. You will time the thirty-second wait before the building can continue if the tower falls.

3. You may not assist the builder or delegator in any way. *Only observe* and time the exercise, which will take a total of three minutes. Call "stop" at the end of three minutes and count the number of cubes in the tower at that point.

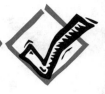

BLIND DELEGATION

INSTRUCTIONS PART B

Directions: Copy and cut apart for participants.

Instructions B: Delegator

1. Plan strategy to be used in building the tower. You have five minutes.
2. Write down the strategy if you wish.
3. Builder is to build as high as possible the tower of singular sugar cubes. Rules are up to the group.
4. Examine the effect that strategy and planning have on the process.

Instructions B: Builder

1. Plan strategy to be used in building the tower. You have five minutes.
2. The goal is to build as high as possible the tower of singular sugar cubes. Continue to wear the blindfold and use your nondominant hand when building. Other rules are up to the group.
3. Examine the effect that strategy and planning have on the process.

Instructions B: Observer

1. Time the strategy session. It is to last five minutes. Tell the group when there are three minutes left and one minute left. Call time.
2. Time the second building attempt for three minutes.
3. When time is called, count the number of cubes in the tower.
4. Share with your delegator and builder the questions handout that is placed on the table by the educator.

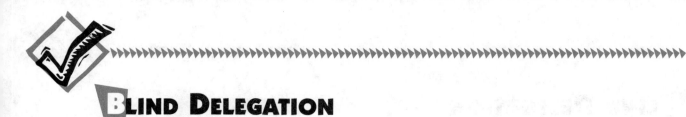

BLIND DELEGATION

QUESTIONS

1. How did you feel in trial A (the first time)?

_____

_____

2. Why do you think thirty seconds was given in between the falling of the tower and rebuilding?

_____

_____

3. What was the outcome the first time?

_____

_____

4. How did you feel in trial B (the second time)?

_____

_____

5. What made the difference and why?

_____

_____

6. How would you apply this information to your work environment?

_____

_____

TOPIC

Teamwork, changing
the paradigm,
problem solving,
delegation

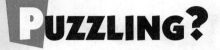

PUZZLING?

TOOL BOX

12–16-piece puzzle,
one per team;
envelopes large
enough to hold
puzzles; watch with
second hand;
discussion questions,
pens or pencils

Preparation

1. Obtain several 12–16-piece children's puzzles. You will need one puzzle per team.
2. Obtain a large brown envelope for each puzzle.
3. Lay the puzzles out one next to each other.
4. Take one piece from puzzle 1 and place it on puzzle 2.
5. Take a piece from puzzle 2 and place it on puzzle 3.
6. Take a piece from puzzle 3 and place it on puzzle 4. Continue this pattern until the last puzzle in the row has its piece placed on top of puzzle 1.
7. Take all the remaining pieces of puzzle 1 and place them on the background cardboard in an envelope with the extra piece.
8. Take all the remaining pieces of puzzle 2 and place them and the background cardboard in an envelope with the extra piece.
9. Continue this pattern until all the puzzles are in envelopes.
10. Obtain a stopwatch and a flipchart to display times as teams complete their puzzles.
11. Make a copy of the question page for each team.
12. Make sure each participant has a pen or pencil.

Implementation

1. Divide your group into teams of two to six people.
2. Introduce to the group the concept of teamwork being a collaborative effort. Tell them this exercise will reinforce the teamwork process.

continued

EDUCATOR SECRETS:

Add all group times
together to show
that the measure
depended on
collaboration.

By: Lanelle C. Picarella, MEd, RN

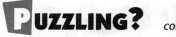 **PUZZLING?** *continued*

3. Hand out one brown envelope per team containing all the puzzle pieces except one, and one piece of another team's puzzle. They will have to go to another team to get the piece they need, but don't tell them this.

4. Tell the teams to work collaboratively to finish the puzzles in the envelopes.

5. Give the signal to open the envelopes and begin. Tell them to applaud wildly when finished.

6. Observe the start time and finish time of each team. Watch how the team members work together, when they realize that they don't have the last piece, and how the teams obtain the last piece they need.

7. Do not get involved in puzzle disputes. Let the teams problem solve.

8. When the teams have finished, give out the discussion questions. Have the teams answer the questions and prepare a team report. Allow about ten minutes for this step.

9. Each team presents one response per question to the entire group.

10. Ask about the paradigm or thought pattern shift, "What happened when you found that the team itself did not have all the pieces to do its puzzle?"

11. Make the point that your team may be a composite member of a larger team. "Collaboration doesn't exist in a closed environment. We may need to shift our paradigm to get the big picture accomplished."

12. Have each person commit to taking some idea back to his or her work team from this presentation.

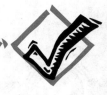

PUZZLING?

QUESTIONS

1. Was there a leader? If so, who?

_____

_____

2. How did the team function together? Did everyone participate?

_____

_____

_____

3. What happened in the team when the last piece didn't fit?

_____

_____

_____

4. How did the team go about finding the last piece?

_____

_____

_____

5. What implications are there for your work team and you?

_____

_____

_____

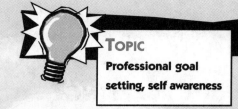

TOOL BOX
A large puzzle (at least 2' x 4') with 1 piece per participant. For a large group, use 8 1/2" x 11" paper to create several smaller puzzles (5–8 pieces), pens or pencils

LOOK AT ME

Preparation

1. Obtain a large puzzle or several smaller ones of five to eight pieces. You can make your own if desired from an 8 1/2" x 11" paper using scissors.

2. Mix the pieces and give out randomly to participants as they enter the room.

3. Make sure that each participant has a pen or pencil.

Implementation

1. If you have a large group, divide the participants into small teams of five to eight people.

2. Explain that the purpose of this activity is to begin to look at who we are as nurses. This activity can be a part of a lecture on professional goal setting.

3. Each participant selects a puzzle piece.

4. Ask each participant to write their response to the question, "The special gifts I bring to nursing are . . . ." on their puzzle piece.

5. If you divided the group into teams, tell the participants to search for the other team members who have matching puzzle pieces.

6. Ask the participants to assemble the puzzle/puzzles.

7. Discuss the uniqueness of each puzzle piece yet how it fits to complete the whole picture.

8. Discuss the unique gifts we bring to our profession and how they fit together to provide quality care.

EDUCATOR SECRETS:
There should be the same number of puzzle pieces as people. If not, present the rest of the puzzle as groups are assembling.

By: Barbara Bonheur, MS, RN

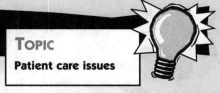

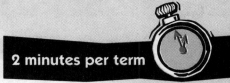

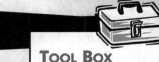

PATIENT CARE PICTURES

Preparation

1. On an index card, write down an appropriate pertinent patient care term for the group. Make several cards, at least six to ten.

2. Obtain a flipchart or write-on board and markers.

3. Locate a timing device or a watch with a second hand.

Implementation

1. The group is divided into two teams; an artist is designated for each team.

2. One team is selected to go first.

3. The artist receives a card with a patient care term written on it.

4. The artist then has one minute to draw a picture describing the patient care term. No words or numbers may be used.

5. If the artist's team does not guess the term, the opposing team gets one chance to guess the term.

6. One point is awarded for each correct response.

7. The teams alternate turns, and at the end of the game, the team with the most points wins.

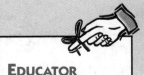

EDUCATOR SECRETS:
Ask for volunteer artists. Don't assign this role. Some feel awkward about their ability to draw.

By: Lana Brumfield, BSN, RN
Nancy Hennen, BSN, RN, C

TOPIC

Any content to review or reinforce

TOOL BOX

Koosh™ ball or super soft object for throwing

KOOSH™ TOSS

Preparation

1. Teach a block of content.
2. Obtain a Koosh™ ball or soft object for throwing. A wadded up sheet of paper can also be used.

Implementation

1. Have everyone stand up and think of at least one point they have learned about the content just presented.
2. Explain the rules for a Koosh™ toss:
   - All throws are underhanded.
   - You must say someone's name and make eye contact before you toss the Koosh™ ball, so that they are ready to catch it.
   - Whoever catches the ball says one thing they have learned today.
   - After they pass the ball to another, they sit down.
   - No one can repeat what another person said.

EDUCATOR SECRETS:

Participate in this activity yourself. Finish by naming something you've learned.

By: Michele Deck, MEd, BSN, RN, ACCE-R
Jeanne Silva, BSN, RN, CCRN

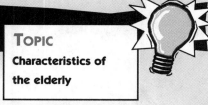
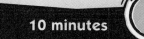

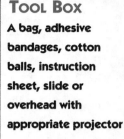

TOOL BOX
A bag, adhesive
bandages, cotton
balls, instruction
sheet, slide or
overhead with
appropriate projector

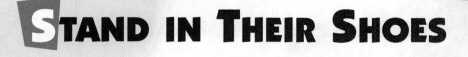

STAND IN THEIR SHOES

Preparation

1. Make several copies of the ready-to-use instruction sheet and cut them into sections.

2. Place the instructions in a bag and mix them up.

3. Obtain some adhesive bandages and cotton balls, and put them where participants may come up and get them.

4. Set up slide or overhead projector with image out of focus.

Implementation

1. Explain to the group that they will experience the characteristics of the elderly firsthand.

2. Have a volunteer pass around the bag of instruction slips. Have each participant take one.

3. Turn on the projector and place the slide or overhead slightly out of focus to simulate vision problems until someone calls your attention to it.

4. Explain this simulates elderly vision.

5. At the end of the time frame, have the learners find a partner and discuss what they have learned by standing in the shoes of an elderly person for three minutes.

6. Debrief important points.

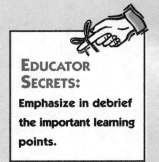

EDUCATOR SECRETS:
Emphasize in debrief the important learning points.

By: Michele Deck, MEd, BSN, RN, ACCE-R
Jeanne Silva, BSN, RN, CCRN

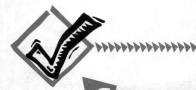

STAND IN THEIR SHOES

LIST OF INSTRUCTIONS

Directions: Cut along rules.

- You are an elderly person. You have suffered a stroke. Write for the next five minutes with your nondominant hand. If your are right-handed, use your left. If your are left-handed, use your right.

- You are an elderly person. Your hearing is failing. Place a small piece of cotton in each ear for the next five minutes.

- You are an elderly person. You have gait and balance problems. Beginning now, place your shoes on the wrong feet. (Place your right shoe on the left foot, and vice versa.) Try to wear your shoes on the wrong feet through the next break and walk slowly and carefully to the restroom. Once you have experienced this walk, you can put them back on properly.

- You are an elderly person. You are experiencing sensation changes in your fingers. Place an adhesive bandage on your right index finger and keep it there until the first break.

TOPIC

Communication. This can also be used to demonstrate differences in charting and assessment skills.

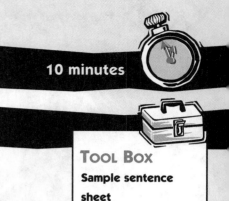

RUMORS!

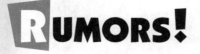

Preparation

1. Copy the ready-to-use sentence sheet.
2. Cut the copy in the space between the two sentences.

Implementation

1. Seat the participants in a circle.
2. Select one participant to start the activity by whispering one of the sample sentences to the participant on his or her right.
3. Explain that the sender of the message must whisper the sentence clearly, but he or she can't repeat the message even if the listener has not heard it.
4. Pass the message around the circle.
5. The last person to receive the message must say it aloud.
6. The original message is then read to the group.
7. A discussion follows with important communication concepts highlighted.

EDUCATOR SECRETS:

Stress important points during the discussion. This is where the learning occurs.

By: Michele Deck, MEd, BSN, RN, ACCE-R
Nancy Hennen, BSN, RNC

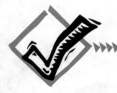

RUMORS!

SAMPLE SENTENCES

"Mrs. Lafayette went to Schwegmann's to buy groceries so she could make gumbo. She bought French bread, rice, okra, andouille sausage, onions, file, chicken, and onions."

"Little Tommy Turnip was a very bad boy. In one day he broke a window, trampled his mother's tulips, tormented a cat, and teased the little red-haired girl next door."

TOPIC

Negative drains and
positive outflows call
on learner creativity

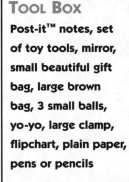

TOOL BOX

Post-it™ notes, set
of toy tools, mirror,
small beautiful gift
bag, large brown
bag, 3 small balls,
yo-yo, large clamp,
flipchart, plain paper,
pens or pencils

It's in the Bag

Preparation

1. Place the Post-it™ notes, toy tools, and mirror in the gift bag.
   Close the gift bag and place it in the bottom of the large brown
   bag. On top of the gift bag, place the balls, yo–yo, and clamp.
   Close the brown bag.

2. Prepare a list of negative drains and positive outflows for the
   audience. This list serves as a reference plus introduction.

3. Make sure each participant has a pen or pencil.

Implementation

1. Tell the audience that at this time our resources are negatively
   drained. Tell them, "We feel clamped down!" Pull out a clamp
   from the bag and display it to the group. "We sometimes feel like
   a yo-yo (or meet yo-yos)." Pull out a yo-yo and play with it at least
   two times. "Or maybe we feel like we're juggling priorities in life."
   Pull out three balls and do a poor job of juggling them.

2. If the group is small, have them voice their negative drains and
   list them on a flipchart. If the group is larger, break into teams and
   have them list their negative drains on a sheet of paper. Team
   leaders report back to the group and copy their lists onto the flipchart.

3. Discuss the importance of identifying negative drains so we know
   where the opportunities for improvement are.

4. Now hold up the brown bag and tear it enough to reveal the
   beautiful gift bag inside. State that "Even though we have drains
   on us, we also have within ourselves positive outflows." Completely
   tear away the brown bag at this point.

5. Pull out the mirror. Ask, "What do you see when you look in the
   mirror? All of us have resources that can be called on individually
   or collectively."

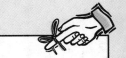

**EDUCATOR
SECRETS:**

Practice ahead of
time tearing the
brown bag away. Put
negative stuff on top
to reach easily.

continued

By: Lanelle C. Picarella, MEd, RN

I T'S IN THE BAG   *continued*

6. Pull out the toy tools. "We may want to use our tools: our talents, experience, and skills. We may need to buy better tools and get more education."

7. Pull out the Post-it™ notes. "Finally, we may want to share our ideas and communicate with others so our positive outflows grow." Pass around the Post-it™ notes and have everyone take one.

8. Ask the group individually or by teams to list the positive outflows on a flipchart. Have them discuss ideas that may counter negative ideas.

9. Discuss the importance of identifying positive outflows individually and as a group so that use of human resources are maximized.

10. Have each participant write down on a Post-it™ note one idea that he or she will take back to the work group on the job to consider.

11. Conclude by saying, "When we apply our positive outflows (hold up gift bag), we can change the negative drains (hold up torn brown bag) into opportunities for creative use of human resources."

TOPIC

Emphasize the fact
the we are better
care givers when
we take care of
ourselves first.

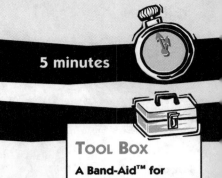

BAND-AID™ REMINDERS

Preparation

1. Obtain a pack of plain or fun Band-Aids™.
2. Teach your content about stress reduction.

Implementation

1. At the completion of a discussion of stress management, ask each participant to think of one thing they have learned that they will commit to implement.
2. Pass out Band-Aids™ and ask everyone to put one on their arm or hand as a reminder to take care of themselves by using a new stress reduction strategy.

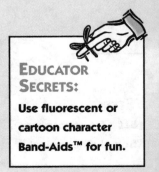

EDUCATOR
SECRETS:

Use fluorescent or
cartoon character
Band-Aids™ for fun.

By: Joanne Ekstedt, BSN, RN, ICCE

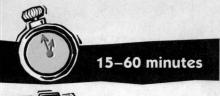
TOPIC

Review just about any topic that has questions to answer. You might ask your learners to write questions and use those.

TOOL BOX

List of questions on subject matter, prize vault, prizes

QUESTION BEE

Preparation

1. Obtain a large box and label it *prize vault*.

2. Place frisbees, cups with tea bags, huggies for soda cans, doodle pads, tote bags, 5th Avenue™ candy bars, and pencil clips in the box.

3. Make up questions about content or plan time for the participants to write the questions.

Implementation

1. Divide the group into two teams.

2. Introduce the prize vault to get them excited about winning. Do not show the prizes, but refer to them by the following abbreviations:

CASH	Circular Aerodynamic Saucer for the Hand (Frisbee™)
TV	Tea Vessel (cup with tea bag)
VCR	Vinyl Cup Receptacle (insulated holder for soda can)
Entertainment Center	Doodle pad
Luggage	Tote bag with hospital logo
Trip to New York	5th Avenue™ candy bar
PC	Pencil Clip

continued

EDUCATOR SECRETS:

Set a fun atmosphere from the beginning!

By: Nancy Yentzen, MS, RNC

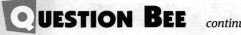

QUESTION BEE *continued*

3. Flip a coin to determine which team begins.

4. Questions are rotated from team to team with only one person answering each time. If the individual's answer is incorrect, the question then goes to the whole team. If the team's answer is incorrect, the opposing team has the opportunity to respond. Scoring: 10 points if the individual answers; 5 points if the team answers; 10 points if the opposing team answers.

5. At the end of the allotted time, scores are tallied.

6. Members on the winning team each select a prize from the list of abbreviations.

7. Actual prizes are awarded after all members have selected items from the list.

TOPIC

Just about any content that can have questions and answers!

TOOL BOX

Flip chart or overhead for an answer board with different points or money amounts in categories, answers to read to groups, small prizes for all, buzzer system

QUESTIONS, NOT ANSWERS

Preparation

1. Develop a number of pertinent questions and answers concerning an important topic or chose a block of content you plan to present.
2. Select the answers and rank them by level of difficulty.
3. Divide the related answers into categories.
4. Assign a point or numeric value to each answer in a category.
5. Turn these categories and point values into an overhead or flipchart.
6. Obtain a buzzer system or some fair way to tell which team has competed to win the first chance to answer.
7. Procure some small, fun prizes or ways to recognize all who participate.

Implementation

1. Divide the group into two or more teams of three to six learners.
2. Explain to team members that they may collaborate on the questions.
3. The instructor will give the answer, and the teams compete to give the question that fits that answer.
4. A team is awarded the points earned when it correctly responds. Points are not deducted if the response is incorrect. The team with the most points at the completion of play wins.

EDUCATOR SECRETS:

Make the selection of the person buzzing in fair, so that everyone will enjoy this activity. Have a second person watch to see who stands first, if you don't have a buzzer system.

By: Cheri Penas, MS, RN, CCRN
Julie Sandstrom, BSN, RN, CCRN

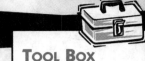

QUESTION TIME!

Preparation

1. Obtain a piece of flipchart paper, and draw a very large question mark on it using colorful markers.
2. Hang this flipchart question mark on the back door of your teaching room.
3. Buy several different colored Post-it™ notes and make them available throughout your teaching area for learners to pick up quickly and easily.
4. Get an attractive party bag or bowl and fill it with small items your learners will like (candy, fruit, Post-it™ notes, pins, etc.).

Implementation

1. Explain to your learners that you have posted a sheet of flipchart paper on the back door of the room.
2. Invite learners if they have a question, to write it down on a Post-it™ note and place it on the poster at breaks and at lunch.
3. Invite everyone to read the questions.
4. Explain that anyone willing to write down an answer on a Post-it™ note may help themselves to a goodie from the bag or bowl.
5. Ask the learners to place the answer next to the question it addresses.
6. Invite all to read the entries at the end of the class.

EDUCATOR SECRETS:

Enlist volunteers to distribute Post-it™ notes. This encourages quiet groups and reluctant learners to participate. Some find peers have more relevant ideas to share than just the instructor.

By: Michele Deck, MEd, BSN, RN, ACCE-R
Jeanne Silva, BSN, RN, CCRN

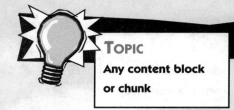

TOOL BOX

Red, yellow, and
green dots stickers

POLKA DOT PAIRS

Preparation

1. Go to an office supply store and buy a large pack of small multicolored dots (they are inexpensive at some of the warehouse type distributors).

2. Cut the sheets up so that each of your learners will have at least five each of the red, yellow, and green dots. If your content is long, give your learners more dots.

Implementation

1. Have the group divide up into pairs.

2. Explain to each pair that they are to review their individual notes on the last block of content.

3. They are to place a green dot next to the areas they feel they understand.

4. They are to place a yellow dot next to any content about which they have questions.

5. They are to place a red dot next to that content that requires further explanation or study.

6. After each learner has taken three to five minutes to place the dots, they are to consult with their partner. If either has a yellow or a red dot, they are to seek out the answers together using the rest of the allotted ten minute time frame. It is possible that one may have a green dot by content that the other has a yellow or red dot on. Encourage students to interact and help each other.

7. The pairs may have to consult a text or another resource person about their red and yellow dots.

8. The duo may plan to follow up with each other two weeks after the class or inservice to make sure that they each understand the material and have begun to implement what they've learned.

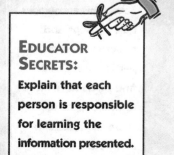

EDUCATOR SECRETS:

Explain that each
person is responsible
for learning the
information presented.

By: Michele Deck, MEd, BSN, RN, ACCE-R
Jeanne Silva, BSN, RN, CCRN

TOPIC

Fear of taking NCLEX exam. This can be adapted for stress reduction, change in the organization, etc.

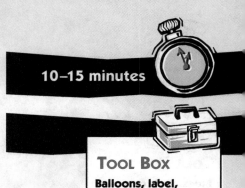

FEARS FLOATING AWAY

Preparation

1. Obtain some colorful helium-filled balloons, one per participant. These are available prefilled or you can purchase the mini party cylinders and fill your own.

2. Gather some colorful thick markers, at least one per participant.

3. Have self-stick colorful name tags or labels ready, at least one per participant.

4. Scout out an outdoor location at your facility that is somewhat private without overhead wires or lines that will interfere with balloon flight.

Implementation

1. Each person is provided with a colorful helium-filled balloon, a label, and a marker.

2. Have each person write down their greatest exam fear or a particular stress factor on the label and stick it on the balloon.

3. They then take the balloons outside and release them.

4. Encourage people to cheer, clap, and celebrate the release of the balloons.

EDUCATOR SECRETS:

Don't fill balloons too early. They can go flat overnight. Use as part of a "pep rally" held for graduate nurses before they take the NCLEX.

By: Sherry Haizlip, BSN, RN, C

TOPIC

Assist those who deal with losses (care of AIDS patients, grief work, etc.) to recognize and deal with their feelings.

DEALING WITH LOSS

Preparation

1. Obtain one 8 1/2" x 11" sheet of paper or ten index cards per participant.

2. Copy your ready-to-use debriefing questions for each participant to use at the end for discussion.

3. Make sure each participant has a pen or pencil.

4. Be aware that this activity may produce high emotional impact for some participants.

Implementation

1. Ask participants to take out a sheet of paper and tear it into ten or fewer pieces (the number of pieces depends on the amount of time you have to do this . . . four is about the minimum). You could also give each person ten index cards.

2. Ask the participants to write down on each card one thing or person which is very important to their life (health, job, spouse, etc.).

3. You then have two options:

   a. Have the participants turn the papers over (like a deck of cards face down) and have the persons to their right pick one. The picker shows the writer what is written on the paper, then tears it up, and throws it away. This thing or person will never exist in the writer's life again. Or . . .

   b. Have the participant read all ten, pick one, look at it, and examine what makes the thing or person special. Have the participant tear it up, and throw it away. This thing or person will never exist in his or her life again. Ask the participants to eliminate another and another.

continued

EDUCATOR SECRETS:

The learning occurs during the debrief of this activity and therefore is *crucial* and can't be omitted.

By: Amanda Martin, MEd, BSN, RN, CNOR

DEALING WITH LOSS *continued*

4. At this point, people get really upset and don't want to play the game or continue. Some people even take out the papers that they don't want to lose.

5. This activity illustrates how people react to loss. It may even get to the point where participants say they would not choose to continue living without some of these essential cards because life isn't worth living without these things or people.

6. This exercise *must* be followed up with a debriefing to discuss feelings, sense of loss, and magnitude and intensity of loss. Distribute the debriefing questions at this time.

7. This activity can be a great springboard for discussion, sharing of personal experiences, and dealing with patients and families in crisis.

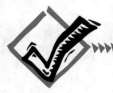

DEALING WITH LOSS

DEBRIEFING QUESTIONS

1. How did you feel when asked to list the ten items most important to you?

2. Did the elimination of the first item surprise you?

3. How does it feel to deal with an unexpected loss?

4. What did you feel when you were told this item was gone forever?

5. Did you want to stop this activity at any point? If so, why?

6. What feelings compelled you to stop?

7. Have you ever observed these types of feelings in others? If so, when?

8. What are some of the coping behaviors you have observed in those experiencing loss?

9. What are some of the situations at work that make us feel this same way?

10. What are some ways we as health care workers can deal with our feelings at times of grief?

11. What are some ways to deal with the frustration we sometimes encounter in our jobs or life?

12. How could you apply what you have learned about loss in this activity to real life?

60–72 minutes

THE CASE OF CREATIVE CRYSTAL VS. DULL AND BORING DAN

Preparation

1. Gather the following supplies: black robe, gavel, prizes relating to the theme of apples or crystal.

2. Make an outline of possible questions for Creative Crystal and Dull and Boring Dan to answer or script a scenario and copy.

3. Have in mind two participants who are not shy and like to be in front of the group.

4. Invite all the participants to bring examples of creative teaching ideas they have used in the past.

Implementation

1. Set the scene as in a courtroom.

2. Ask participants to serve on the jury in the case of Creative Crystal (a teacher who uses creative techniques) and Dull and Boring Dan (a teacher who uses traditional methods). The instructor or a volunteer can act as judge.

3. Participants hear testimony about how Crystal uses games and simulations, case studies, and role plays to enhance the effectiveness of educational programming.

4. Along with testimony from Crystal, select a few of the audience members to testify about creative ideas. They must bring a creative teaching idea to class to discuss and/or demonstrate. Dan talks about how bored his participants are in class and demonstrates his lecture based teaching technique.

5. The jury votes on the most creative teaching technique shared with the court.

6. Everyone who participates gets a prize.

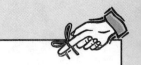

EDUCATOR SECRETS:
You might want to prearrange who will testify or demonstrate so that they have the necessary props, etc.

By: Phyllis J. Miller, MS, RN, FHCE

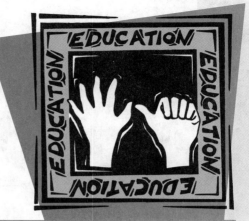

PART 4

INSTANT TOOLS FOR CURRICULUM AND CONTINUING EDUCATION

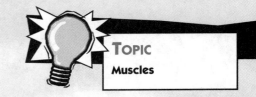
TOOL BOX

Those Amazing
Muscles Match Game,
pens or pencils,
answer key

THOSE AMAZING MUSCLES

Preparation

1. Make a copy of the ready-to-use Those Amazing Muscles match game for each participant.

2. Make sure each participant has a pen or pencil.

3. Use this activity as a preassessment or introduction before the lesson or as a review after the lesson.

4. Make a copy of the answer key.

Implementation

1. Ask the learners, individually or in teams of two to six, to match the correct muscle with its description.

2. Recruit volunteers to share their answers with the entire group.

3. Clarify any needed points.

4. Extra idea: If your group is reviewing, invite learners to turn in the completed sheets. Use the sheets as an entry to a prize drawing the next day.

EDUCATOR SECRETS:

Ask the learners to mark on the picture at the bottom of the page each muscle as they match it.

By: Nancy Hennen, BSN, RNC

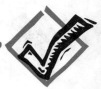

THOSE AMAZING MUSCLES MATCH GAME

Directions: Match the correct muscle with its description.

1. This muscle delivers a knockout punch. _____

2. This muscle helps you kick a ball. _____

3. This muscle allows you to stand on tiptoe. _____

4. This muscle shows how strong you are. _____

5. When this tendon is cut, it is hard to walk. _____

6. This muscle helps you raise your arm. _____

7. This muscle group helps you kneel. _____

8. This is the muscle that the bodybuilders are so proud of. _____

9. These diamond-shaped muscles cover the back of the neck and shoulders. _____

10. This is your natural shoulder pad. _____

Key Terms
Pectoralis
Trapezius
Deltoid
Biceps
Triceps
Serratus
Quadriceps
Hamstring
Gastrocnemius
Achilles tendon

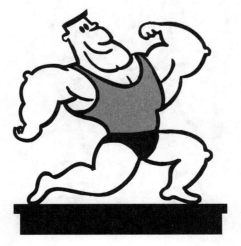

THOSE AMAZING MUSCLES MATCH GAME

ANSWER KEY

Directions: Match the correct muscle with its description.

1. This muscle delivers a knockout punch. <u>Triceps</u>

2. This muscle helps you kick a ball. <u>Quadriceps</u>

3. This muscle allows you to stand on tiptoe. <u>Gastrocnemius</u>

4. This muscle shows how strong you are. <u>Biceps</u>

5. When this tendon is cut, it is hard to walk. <u>Achilles tendon</u>

6. This muscle helps you raise your arm. <u>Serratus</u>

7. This muscle group helps you kneel. <u>Hamstring</u>

8. This is the muscle that the bodybuilders are so proud of. <u>Pectoralis</u>

9. These diamond-shaped muscles cover the back of the neck and shoulders. <u>Trapezius</u>

10. This is your natural shoulder pad. <u>Deltoid</u>

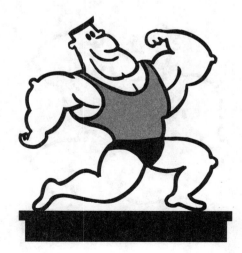

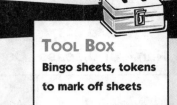

TOOL BOX

Bingo sheets, tokens to mark off sheets

NCLEX BINGO

Preparation

1. Make a copy of the ready-to-use NCLEX bingo sheet for each participant.
2. Copy the clue sheet. Cut this up for bingo pulls.

Implementation

1. Poll the group to see how many people are familiar with the game of bingo.
2. Explain that NCLEX appears at the top of the grid rather than BINGO.
3. Have the learners pay attention to this detail: the initials of the column heads are significant. The *N* column is the *N*ames of diseases, the *C* is for *C*omplications, the *L* is for *L*ab values, the *E* is for *E*xamination results, and the *X* is for e*X*tra trivia facts.
4. Offer the learners a chance to alter their cards. The N and the E columns have alternate descriptions at the bottom of the column. The learners may replace the information in any box in those columns with an alternate from the bottom.
5. Now play bingo, calling out clues randomly. For example, say, "Under the E, these are the examination findings in a patient with thrombophlebitis. Please mark off the box that corresponds to thrombophlebitis."
6. Invite the first person with bingo horizontally, vertically, diagonally, or with the four corners to stand. He or she is the winner.
7. Play as many games as it takes to reinforce the information.

EDUCATOR SECRETS:

Enlist volunteers to hand out the sheets for you.

By: Michele Deck, MEd, BSN, RN, ACCE-R
Jeanne Silva, BSN, RN, CCRN

NCLEX BINGO

N C L E X

N Name of Disease	**C** Complications	**L** Labs	**E** Examinations	**X** X-tras
MI	Anxiety, dyspnea, rapid onset, complication r/t surgery or immobility, often has hemoptysis	↑ BUN ↑ Creatinine ↑ Potassium ↓ Sodium	SOB, peripheral edema, rales, CVP elevated	Defibrillate or Check patient or Call a code
Acute renal failure	Seen in patients with a longstanding history of hypertension	↑ CPK ↑ MB	↑ Calf size, tenderness, swelling and + Homan's	OSHA guidelines
CVA	A febrile infection seen in surgery patients who don't have respiratory therapy treatments and don't cough and deep breathe	**FREE**	Temp/chills, productive cough, tachycardia, percussion dullness, ↓ breath sounds	CPR
Diabetes mellitus	Patients in ICU settings can have this complication. Signs include stools positive for blood, decreasing H&H	↓ Platelets ↓ WBC	Pain (chest, jaw, arm, back), nausea, vomiting diaphoresis, SOB, ECG changes	Last day of state board exams
Hodgkin's disease	Patients who are immunosuppressed or have low PLT/WBC are highly susceptible to this	↑ AST ↑ ALT ↑ Bilirubin	↓ H&H, + Guiac stool, food intolerance, hematemesis	One to two years depending on the state you live in
Peptic ulcer			Headache, vision disturbances, pupil changes, changes in LOC	

NCLEX BINGO CLUES

Under the N Clues:

 Occlusion of one or more coronary arteries causing death of a portion of the myocardial tissue (*MI*)

 A sudden and potentially reversible loss of kidney function (*Acute renal failure*)

N Severe, sudden decrease in cerebral circulation caused by either a thrombus or hemorrhage resulting in a cerebral infarct (*CVA*)

N A chronic systemic disease producing disorder in carbohydrate, protein, and fat metabolism; results from disturbances in the production, action, or use of insulin (*Diabetes mellitus*)

N Malignancy of the lymphoid system characterized by a generalized, painless lymphadenopathy (*Hodgkin's disease*)

N Sharply defined break in mucosa, which may involve the submucosa and muscular layers of the esophagus, stomach, and duodenum (*Peptic ulcer*)

Under the C Clues:

C Pulmonary embolus (*Anxiety, dyspnea, rapid onset, complication r/t surgery or immobility, often has hemoptysis*)

C Pneumonia (*A febrile infection seen in surgery patients who don't have respiratory treatments and don't cough and deep breathe.*)

C Peptic ulcer (*Patients located in ICU settings can have this complication. Signs include stools positive for blood, decreasing H&H*)

C Sepsis (*Patients who are immunosuppressed or have low PLT/WBC are highly susceptible to this*)

C Renal failure (*Seen in patients with a longstanding history of hypertension*)

Under the L Clues:

 Acute renal failure (*Increased BUN, increased creatinine, increased potassium, decreased sodium*)

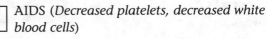 MI
(*Increased CPK, increased MB*)

L AIDS (*Decreased platelets, decreased white blood cells*)

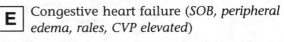 Liver disease (*Increased AST, increased ALT, increased bilirubin*)

Under the E Clues:

E Congestive heart failure (*SOB, peripheral edema, rales, CVP elevated*)

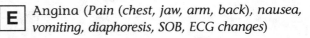 Thrombophlebitis (*Increased calf size, tenderness, swelling, + Homans'*)

E Pneumonia (*Temp/chills, productive cough, tachycardia, percussion dullness, decreased breath sounds*)

 Angina (*Pain (chest, jaw, arm, back), nausea, vomiting, diaphoresis, SOB, ECG changes*)

E Peptic ulcer (*Decreased H&H, + Guiac stool, food intolerance, hematemesis*)

E Increased intracranial pressure (*Headache, vision disturbances, pupil changes, changes in LOC*)

Under the X Clues:

 The appropriate first response to a cardiac monitor that shows ventricular tachycardia at a rate of 170/minute (*Check the patient*)

 These say that one cannot eat, drink, apply makeup, remove or insert contact lenses in patient areas (*OSHA guidelines*)

 ABCs are done for this
(*CPR*)

X The day that all NCLEX takers have a blow out party (*Last day of state board exams*)

 How often you must renew your nursing license (*One to two years depending on the state you live in*)

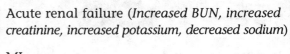
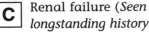

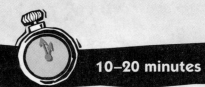

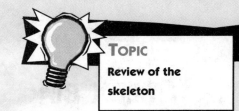

TOOL BOX

Dem Bones crossword puzzle, pens or pencils, answer key

DEM BONES CROSSWORD PUZZLE

Preparation

1. Make a copy of the ready-to-use Dem Bones crossword puzzle for each participant.

2. Use this as an introduction to the lesson or as a review after the lesson.

3. Make sure each participant has a pen or pencil.

4. Make a copy of the answer key.

Variation

1. Use a poster printer copy machine to turn the crossword into a poster-size image.

2. Plan for groups of two to six to discuss and fill in a poster-size copy of the crossword puzzle before or after your lesson.

Implementation

1. Pass out the large or small crossword puzzle.

2. Challenge your learners to complete the puzzle as individuals or as teams.

3. If energy and attention are low during your lesson presentation, stop and let your participants engage in this energizing activity.

4. Crossword puzzles can also be sent out days or weeks after the lsson as reinforcement of important concepts.

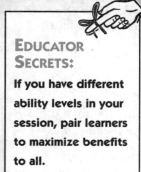

EDUCATOR SECRETS:

If you have different ability levels in your session, pair learners to maximize benefits to all.

By: Amanda Martin, MEd, BSN, RN, CNOR

DEM BONES CROSSWORD PUZZLE

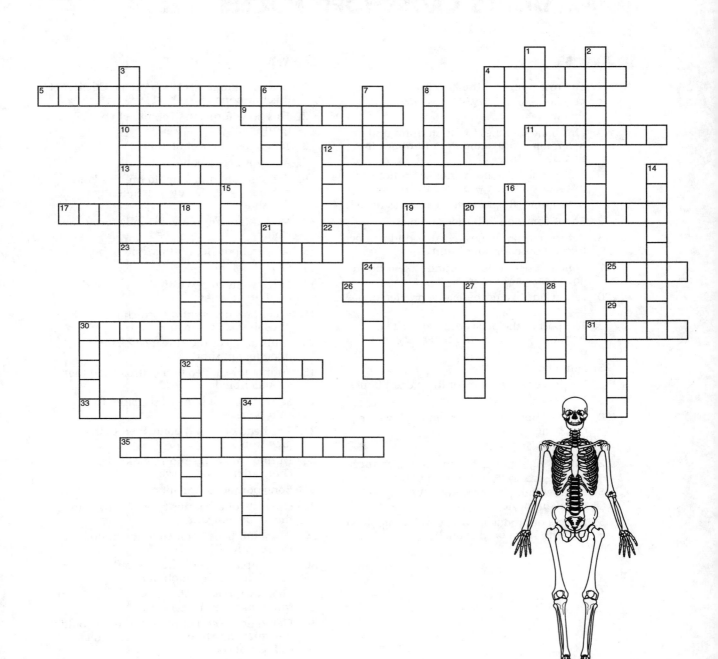

continued

DEM BONES CROSSWORD PUZZLE *continued*

Across

4. The real name for the kneecap
5. Soft, spongy bone (You "can" remember this stuff)
9. This bone attaches to the sternum and acromion process and lies just above the first rib
10. This pelvic bone has winglike portions to rest kids on when you hold them
11. Breastbone; the bone you compress in CPR
12. Bones common to hands and feet
13. Put the cranial bones together and you get this; a house for your brain
17. Bone of upper arm; it sounds like it has a good sense of humor
20. Femur has two of these: one greater, one lesser
22. The part of the pelvis that you "sit" on. Actually, you sit on the tuberosity part of it
23. Hand bones
25. You have twelve pairs of these chest bones
26. Foot bones
30. A little "untruthful" bone in the lower leg; calf bone
31. You have 206 of these
32. Ninety-eight percent of the body's extracellular _____ is in bones; a mineral
33. Marrow that produces RBCs, WBCs, and megakaryocytes
35. Process of producing and developing blood cells (no hints on this one!)

Down

1. Low calcium levels stimulate production of this hormone
2. This bone forms the "point" of your elbow (part of ulna)
3. Tough, outer cover of bones
4. Anterior pelvic bone
6. The sternum and scapula are this kind of bone; Wiley Coyote is frequently in this shape
7. Medial forearm bone; actually forms the elbow
8. Shape of patella; it's this kind of bone
12. Elvis shook his
14. These come in cervical, thoracic, and lumbar varieties
15. Facilitates absorption of calcium and phosphorus (2 words)
16. Arms and legs are classified as this type of bone; not short
18. Triangular-shaped bone; also called the shoulder blade
19. Second longest bone in skeleton; the shin bone
21. The head of a long bone; next to the growth plate
24. During stress, this marrow may be changed into red marrow
27. Bone parallel to the ulna
28. Opposite of long; this type of bone is in the ankle and wrist
29. Your "tail bone"; joined to the bottom of the sacrum
30. "The hip bone is connected to the thigh bone"; this is the thigh bone
32. This is what you call the hard, dense bone that makes up the bone shaft
34. Found at the end of the sternum; it could puncture something if hand placement for CPR is not correct

DEM BONES CROSSWORD PUZZLE

ANSWER KEY

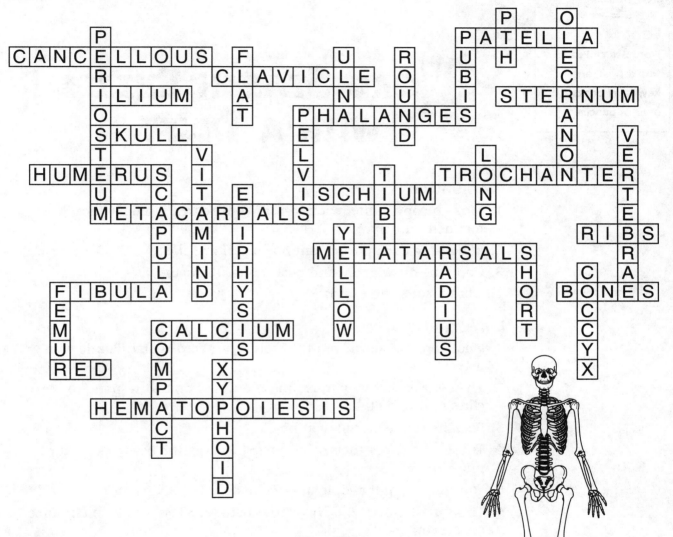

Across

4. Patella
5. Cancellous
9. Clavicle
10. Ilium
11. Sternum
12. Phalanges
14. Skull
17. Humerus
20. Trochanter
22. Ischium
23. Metacarpals
25. Ribs
26. Metatarsals
30. Fibula
31. Bones
32. Calcium
33. Red
35. Hematopoiesis

Down

1. PTH
2. Olecranon
3. Periosteum
4. Pubis
6. Flat
7. Vina
8. Round
12. Pelvis
14. Vertebrae
15. Vitamin D
16. Long
18. Scapula
19. Tibia
20. Epiphysis
24. Yellow
27. Radius
28. Short
29. Coccyx
31. Femur
33. Compact
34. Xiphoid

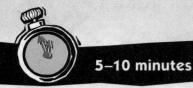
TOOL BOX

Word Search Puzzle
with a Twist, answer
key, small prizes,
pens or pencils

WORD SEARCH PUZZLE WITH A TWIST

Preparation

1. Make a copy of the ready-to-use Word Search Puzzle with a Twist for each participant.
2. Make sure each participant has a pen or pencil.
3. Copy the answer key and post it after the activity.
4. Obtain some small prizes.

Implementation

1. Challenge the participants to solve the Word Search Puzzle with a Twist.
2. The twist is that they must find the words that correspond to the clues and circle them.
3. Post the results at the next break.
4. Those who check their answers first will get the best pick of the prizes.
5. You can also put people in pairs to do this activity.
6. This puzzle can also be given out between classes to help reinforce course content.

EDUCATOR SECRETS:

Review and reinforce content in a fun, interactive way!

By: Michele Deck, MEd, BSN, RN, ACCE-R
Jeanne Silva, BSN, RN, CCRN

WORD SEARCH PUZZLE WITH A TWIST

Directions: Circle the words that correspond to the definitions below. Words may appear forward, backward, up, or down.

```
K  S  G  N  I  H  S  U  C  T  S
C  J  L  U  P  U  S  S  O  R  E
O  F  A  S  M  I  L  D  Q  U  P
H  D  U  R  E  F  X  I  H  L  I
S  T  C  A  R  A  T  A  C  I  L
B  D  O  W  A  N  I  G  N  A  E
H  E  M  O  R  R  H  O  I  D  P
S  H  A  R  T  H  R  I  T  I  S
C  I  R  R  H  O  S  I  S  K  Y
```

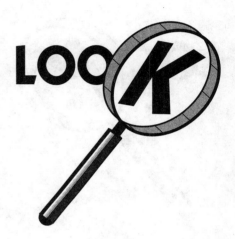

1. A syndrome associated with abnormal cellular metabolism; the pathology is inadequate tissue perfusion

2. Chest pain caused by temporary ischemia of the myocardium; usually caused by atherosclerosis, arteriosclerosis, thrombus, or coronary spasm

3. Chronic degenerative disease of the liver causing inflammation, destruction, fibrotic regeneration, and hepatic insufficiency

4. Excessive secretion of glucocorticoids and possibly androgens from the adrenal cortex

5. Dilated vein under the mucous membranes in the anal area; may be internal or external

6. Episode of uncontrolled electrical activity in the brain; neuronal discharges become excessive and irregular, resulting in loss of consciousness, convulsive body movements, or disturbances in sensation or behavior

7. Total or partial opacity of the normally transparent crystalline lens; the opacity of the lens interferes with light passage through the lens

8. Abnormal increase in intraocular pressure caused by any obstruction of the outflow channels of aqueous humor

9. A chronic, systemic, diffuse, collagen disease characterized by inflammatory changes in joints and related structures, resulting in crippling deformities

10. Generalized connective tissue disorder; difficult to diagnose, with no cure

11. Syndrome characterized by a defect in cell mediated immunity; may have a long incubation period

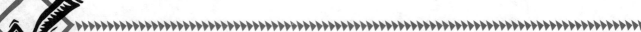

WORD SEARCH PUZZLE WITH A TWIST

ANSWER KEY

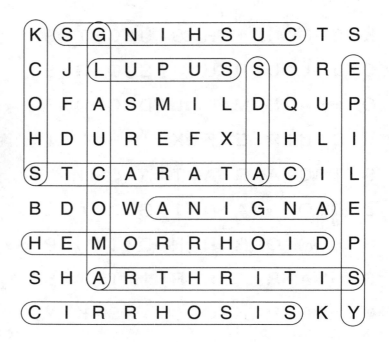

```
K  S  G  N  I  H  S  U  C  T  S
C  J  L  U  P  U  S  S  O  R  E
O  F  A  S  M  I  L  D  Q  U  P
H  D  U  R  E  F  X  I  H  L  I
S  T  C  A  R  A  T  A  C  I  L
B  D  O  W  A  N  I  G  N  A  E
H  E  M  O  R  R  H  O  I  D  P
S  H  A  R  T  H  R  I  T  I  S
C  I  R  R  H  O  S  I  S  K  Y
```

LOOK

1. A syndrome associated with abnormal cellular metabolism; the pathology is inadequate tissue perfusion *(shock)*

2. Chest pain caused by temporary ischemia of the myocardium; usually caused by atherosclerosis, arteriosclerosis, thrombus, or coronary spasm *(angina)*

3. Chronic degenerative disease of the liver causing inflammation, destruction, fibrotic regeneration, and hepatic insufficiency *(cirrhosis)*

4. Excessive secretion of glucocorticoids and possibly androgens from the adrenal cortex *(Cushing's)*

5. Dilated vein under the mucous membranes in the anal area; may be internal or external *(hemorrhoid)*

6. Episode of uncontrolled electrical activity in the brain; neuronal discharges become excessive and irregular, resulting in loss of consciousness, convulsive body movements, or disturbances in sensation or behavior *(epilepsy)*

7. Total or partial opacity of the normally transparent crystalline lens; the opacity of the lens interferes with light passage through the lens *(cataracts)*

8. Abnormal increase in intraocular pressure caused by any obstruction of the outflow channels of aqueous humor *(glaucoma)*

9. A chronic, systemic, diffuse, collagen disease characterized by inflammatory changes in joints and related structures, resulting in crippling deformities *(arthritis)*

10. Generalized connective tissue disorder; difficult to diagnose, with no cure *(lupus)*

11. Syndrome characterized by a defect in cell mediated immunity; may have a long incubation period *(AIDS)*

TOPIC

This exercise is used to help RNs become more proficient in using nursing diagnoses.

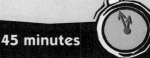

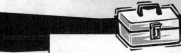

45 minutes

Is It or Isn't It?

TOOL BOX

30–40 index cards with nursing diagnoses; treatments; medical diagnoses; and cards that say, "Pass a card to the player to your left (right, across from you, etc.)"; NANDA list, small prize

Preparation

1. Obtain thirty to forty index cards.
2. Obtain the NANDA Nursing Diagnosis list, and make a copy for each participant and for yourself.
3. Choose the nursing diagnoses you plan to utilize from the NANDA list.
4. Write selected nursing diagnoses on twenty to thirty cards.
5. Write four selected *medical* diagnoses on four cards.
6. Write four treatments on four cards.
7. Write a card that says, "Pass a card to the player on your left," "Pass a card to the player on your right," "Pass a card to the player across from you," and "Pass a card to any player."
8. Collect some simple prizes or goodies.

Implementation

1. Explain that the objective is to have the most cards at the end.
2. The first player turns a card over and reads it aloud.
3. The player must state if it is or is not a *nursing* diagnosis.
4. If it is a nursing diagnosis and the player says it is, then he or she keeps the card.

   For example, CHF *medical* diagnosis becomes fluid volume excess *nursing* diagnosis.
5. If the player doesn't know if the card lists a nursing diagnosis, the card gets passed to the next person to try. Players are allowed to have the most recent NANDA Nursing Diagnosis list in front of them.
6. The play continues until all cards are completed or time runs out.
7. The person with the most cards gets a small reward.

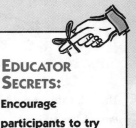

By: Raeleen Roberts, MSN, RN, CCRN

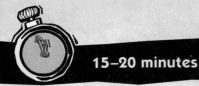

TOOL BOX
Paper, tape, and pen. Name tags can substitute for paper and tape.

TOPIC
Interpretation of dysrhythmia. This can be adapted to any condition with characteristics or symptoms.

NAME THAT RHYTHM

Preparation

1. Write down the names of dysrhythmias on paper or name tags.

Implementation

1. Tape the dysrhythmia names on the learners' backs. The learners cannot see the names on their backs.

2. Explain that the goal is to get the learners to guess the name of the dysrhythmia on their backs by asking questions from the other learners in class. The participants can respond to questions with a *yes, no,* or *maybe.*

3. Model this activity. For example, "Is my heart rate greater than 100?" Response: "No. "Are the P waves before every QRS?" Response: "No."

4. The object of the activity is to have everyone guess which dysrhythmia is on his or her back.

5. Once they have correctly guessed their own, they move the paper to their front and continue to answer questions for those yet to guess.

EDUCATOR SECRETS:
The educator should model the activity once so that the learners understand the process.

By: Kim Major Walker, MSN, RN, CCRN

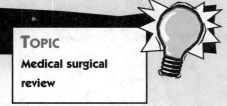

TOOL BOX
Name tags, list of
medical conditions

I'VE GOT A SECRET!

Preparation

1. Obtain name tags, one per participant.
2. Make a copy of the ready-to-use list of medical conditions for each participant.

Implementation

1. Divide the group into teams of four.
2. Distribute a blank name tag to each learner.
3. Ask participants to select a condition from the master list and write it on the name tag without showing it to anyone.
4. Invite the participants to peel and stick the name tag on the back of one of their team members without letting that person see what is says.
5. Each person can then ask *yes*-or-*no* questions to discover what condition is on his or her back. Only *yes* or *no* responses are allowed.
6. The object is to have everyone guess his or her condition correctly.
7. Once the secret condition is discovered, the learner removes the name tag from his or her back and places it on his or her front.

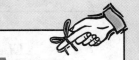

EDUCATOR SECRETS:
This activity can also be adapted to content covered in the lesson by putting main concepts on name tags.

By: Michele Deck, MEd, BSN, RN, ACCE-R
Jeanne Silva, BSN, RN, CCRN

I've Got a Secret!

MEDICAL CONDITIONS

myocardial infarct	congestive heart failure
hypertension	COPD
cholelithiasis	pancreatitis
hepatitis	hypothyroid
cystitis	Crohn's disease
myasthenia gravis	parkinsonism
meningitis	multiple sclerosis
benign prostatic hypertrophy (BHP)	diverticulitis
tuberculosis	hiatal hernia
systemic lupus erythematosus (SLE)	ruptured disk

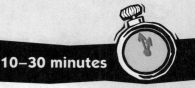

10–30 minutes

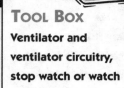
TOPIC
Ways to improve
psychomotor skills
and speed with
assembling ventilator
circuits. This idea can
be adapted to use
with any new
equipment or
technology.

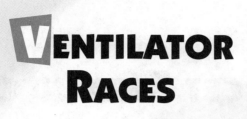

VENTILATOR RACES

Preparation

1. Assemble the needed equipment for ventilator circuit.
2. Decide whether you will use a watch with a second hand or a stop watch.

Implementation

1. To increase the skill and confidence of learners handling ventilator circuitry and to decrease the amount of time to assemble the circuits, students should first practice this activity.
2. Once there has been adequate practice time, play beat the clock in putting the ventilators together.
3. Set up teams and have each member compete to set the circuit up correctly as quickly as possible. Individual times are added to get team times.
4. A twist on this is to set up the circuit incorrectly, asking the learners to troubleshoot the problem and fix it. This gives them the opportunity to use assessment skills. The educator can see how long it takes the learners to problem solve.
5. The learners can also set up a situation for other team members to troubleshoot. This encourages growth of critical thinking skills.

EDUCATOR SECRETS:
Give teams adequate
practice time before
competing, and
equalize skill levels
in small groups.
Individuals can race
against their own
best times to
improve.

By: Mary LaBiche, MEd, RRT

TOOL BOX

Target poster, markers, flash cards with terminology, definition card sets

TARGET TERMINOLOGY

Preparation

1. Divide the medical terms into prefixes, roots, suffixes, and abbreviations.

2. Make colored flash cards with a specific type of term on a specific color. Example: prefixes on red cards and roots on orange cards.

3. Copy the sheets of complete definitions so that each participant has one.

4. Make a flipchart page with a large target on it, so that scores can be posted throughout the activity. The bands or rings of the target should have a correlation to the number of terms used in this activity.

5. Make some markers to place on the target, one for each participant or team.

Implementation

1. Choose one category (prefix, root, suffix, abbreviation) to begin.

2. Complete one category at a time.

3. The instructor holds up a flash card so that all participants can view it. The flash card displays the term to be defined.

4. All participants have a complete set of definitions for each category in front of them on cards. They have ten seconds to find the correct definition and raise their hands.

5. Everyone who selects the appropriate definition is awarded a point.

continued

EDUCATOR SECRETS:

Encourage learners to participate. Put people in twos or threes to play.

By: Michele Deck, MEd, BSN, RN, ACCE-R
Nancy Hennen, BSN, RNC

TARGET TERMINOLOGY *continued*

6. Points are tallied after each question, and a running score is posted on a picture of a target. As points are accumulated, a marker is used to move toward the "Bull's Eye of Correct Medical Terminology."

7. The participants are rewarded by seeing their progress displayed on the target.

8. THUNDER ROUND. This is used for a quick review of medical terminology. All players start by standing up. When they miss a term, they sit down and observe. The last person standing wins. (Similar to a spelling bee)

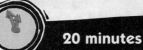
TOOL BOX

Art and Prudent Art cartoons, overhead projector, dry erase pens, answer key

TOPIC

Review the signs and symptoms of a heart attack and appropriate interventions. Any other topic that has humorous cartoon representations can be used.

CARDIAC CARTOON CAPERS

Preparation

1. Make a transparency of both of the ready-to-use cartoons.

2. Set up an overhead projector. Obtain dry erase pens to write on the overhead transparencies.

3. Make enough copies of the cartoons to give half the class Art and the other half Prudent Art.

4. Make a copy of the cartoons and the answer key for yourself.

Implementation

1. Tell the group that the purpose is to review the signs and symptoms of a heart attack and the appropriate interventions. Divide the group into teams of three to five people. The teams work together and use any resource books they have with them.

2. Give each member of a team the same cartoon, making sure that half the teams get one cartoon and half the other.

3. Instruct the teams to read their stories and label the cartoon with the signs and symptoms of a heart attack. Allow time for the teams to work.

4. List the appropriate interventions after the teams have completed their cartoons.

5. Review using the overhead transparency. Bring out the differences in management of MI symptoms in someone with known heart disease.

6. Clarify, explain, or recap the important information as needed.

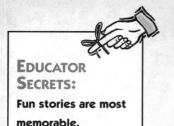

EDUCATOR SECRETS:

Fun stories are most memorable.

By: Barbara Bonheur, MS, RN

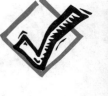

CARDIAC CARTOON CAPERS

THE STORY OF ART

Art A. Tack is fifty-five years old. He smokes a pack of cigarettes a day and, as you can see, is a little overweight. His idea of exercise is getting up to find the TV remote. At his recent check-up, his blood pressure was 142/98 and his cholesterol was 310. He thought the numbers might mean something so he played the lottery with them and won! But his luck is about to change. Art is about to have his first cardiac arrest.

Here's a picture of him moments before the fateful event. See if you can identify the early warning signs.

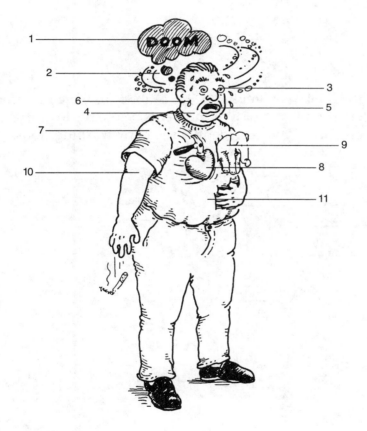

You, thinking quickly, take the following actions:

1._____

2._____

3._____

4._____

155

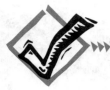

CARDIAC CARTOON CAPERS

THE STORY OF PRUDENT ART

Prudent Art is sixty-five years old. Ten years ago you saved his life when he had a cardiac arrest, and in gratitude, he split his lottery winnings with you. Since then, Art has been into prudent heart living. He is a slim, trim, active, nonsmoker. He has also started raising alligators as a pastime to decrease stress. He still occasionally has angina and takes nitroglycerine.

Today, he came home to find his favorite alligator, Fred, missing and a note that read:

> Dear Prudent Art,
>
> I have decided to move to Florida where the gators go wild.
>
> See ya later alligator

Prudent Art is distraught beyond limits. He is about to have his *second* heart attack. Here is a picture of him moments before his fateful *second* heart event. See if you can identify the early warning signs.

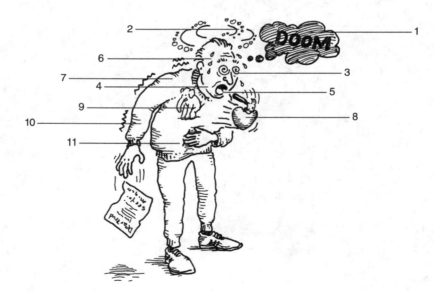

You, thinking quickly, take the following actions:

1._____

2._____

3._____

4._____

CARDIAC CARTOON CAPERS

ANSWER KEY

If you are still wondering what signs and symptoms Art and Prudent Art are experiencing, they are from head down:

1. Cloud of doom
2. Light-headedness (bubbles)
3. Dizziness (eyes swirling)
4. Jaw pain
5. Denial statement ("Don't worry. It's just indigestion.")
6. Sweat
7. Shoulder pain
8. Pounding heart (a hammer pounding)
9. Crushing chest pain (an elephant sitting on the chest)
10. Arm pain
11. Nausea (It's a green stomach on the overhead.)

You, acting quickly, take the following actions:

Art (No History of Heart Disease)	Prudent Art (Known Heart Disease)
1. Recognize	1. Recognize
2. Rest and Reassure	2. Rest and Reassure
3. Wait two minutes	3. Nitroglycerine q. 3–5' (x3)
4. Dial 911 PRN	4. Dial 911 PRN

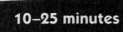

TOPIC

Review cardiopul-
monary circulation.
This can also be used
to show system
physiology or flow
relationship.

TOOL BOX

Plastic hats or visors,
light blue and bright
red paper hearts,
cardiopulmonary
circulation diagram.

HEART HATS

Preparation

1. Create fifteen Heart Hats (these are plastic hats or visors that have a heart attached to the front, each heart listing a step in cardiopulmonary circulation). Color code the hats so that the steps that involve clean, fresh air coming in are light blue and the steps in which oxygen-rich blood gets to the body are bright red.

2. Obtain a diagram of cardiopulmonary circulation large enough to use as an instructional aid.

Implementation

1. Teach or review cardiopulmonary circulation as needed.

2. Distribute one heart hat to each of the fifteen participants.

3. Explain that each heart lists a step in cardiopulmonary circulation.

4. Direct the group to put on their heart hats and to line up from left to right so that the steps to circulation are in order.

5. The educator must review for accuracy, making corrections as needed.

6. Instruct the group that the hearts have been color coded.
   light blue = clean, fresh air coming in
   bright red = steps in which oxygen-rich blood gets to the body

7. Review the circulation process chunking the information by asking similar colors to stand together.

8. Ask the participants to switch heart hats and reorganize the line so that the steps of circulation are in order.

9. Review for accuracy.

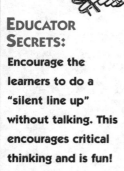

**EDUCATOR
SECRETS:**

Encourage the
learners to do a
"silent line up"
without talking. This
encourages critical
thinking and is fun!

By: Barbara Bonheur, MS, RN

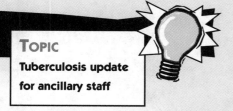

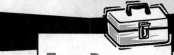
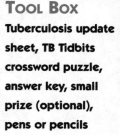

TOOL BOX
Tuberculosis update
sheet, TB Tidbits
crossword puzzle,
answer key, small
prize (optional),
pens or pencils

TB TIDBITS CROSSWORD PUZZLE

Preparation

1. Make copies of the ready-to-use Tuberculosis Update sheet and TB Tidbits crossword puzzle for each participant.

2. Make a copy of the answer key.

3. Collect some small prize or giveaway.

4. Make sure each participant has a pen or pencil.

Implementation

1. Introduce the topic to your learners.

2. Present the information on the update sheet orally or have the participants read it individually.

3. Challenge your learners to complete the crossword puzzle.

4. Offer a prize in a drawing of all correctly completed puzzles or just enjoy this activity because it is energizing and fun.

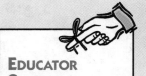

EDUCATOR
SECRETS:
Post the results of
the crossword puzzle
for self checks.

By: Nancy Hennen, BSN, RNC

TUBERCULOSIS UPDATE

The Rise of TB!

In case you haven't heard, the number of TB cases in the United States is on the rise. From 1985 to 1991 the number of reported TB cases jumped 18.4 percent. Most alarming, a growing percentage of these new cases of TB are resistant to the drugs that are traditionally used to fight the disease.

Who Is at Risk?

- HIV-infected persons
- Close contacts of persons with active infectious TB
- Persons with conditions that increase the risk of active TB after infection (DM, chronic renal failure, malignancies, etc.)
- Persons born in countries with a high prevalence of TB
- Substance abusers, such as alcoholics, IV drug users, and cocaine or crack users
- Residents of long-term care facilities, nursing homes, prisons, mental institutions, homeless shelters, and other congregate housing settings
- Medically underserved low-income populations
- Health care workers and others who provide service to any high-risk group

How Is TB Transmitted?

- TB is transmitted when another person inhales a droplet nuclei emitted by an infected person while coughing, sneezing, speaking, or singing.
- It is not transmitted through contact with such things as clothing, bedding, food, or eating utensils as was once believed.
- It is not easily transmitted. Most people exposed to TB don't become infected.
- The body's first line of defense, the upper airway, prevents most inhaled TB organisms from ever reaching the lungs.

Signs and Symptoms of TB?

- Persistent or productive cough
- Weight loss
- Anorexia
- Fever
- Night sweats
- Fatigue
- Undiagnosed pulmonary disease

Infection Control Guidelines:

Be suspicious of any high-risk individual with signs and symptoms of TB
- Facilitate diagnostic testing (AFB smears and cultures, CXR)
- Place patient on "Respiratory Isolation"
- Provide isolation rooms
- Source control
  - Have patient cover mouth to cough, etc.
  - Use particulate respirator masks, taped outside the patient's door, when patient is TB positive
  - Decontamination of items properly
- Systematically screen health care personnel (TB skin test)

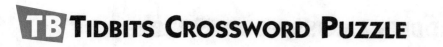

TB TIDBITS CROSSWORD PUZZLE

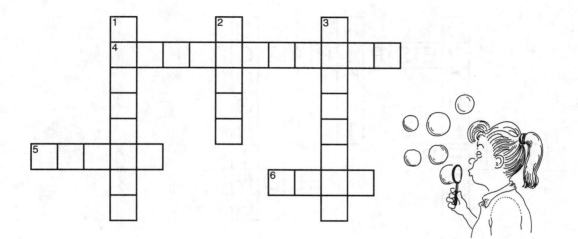

Across

4. In what type of isolation do you place a patient with active infectious TB?

5. The first line of defense against TB is the _____ airway

6. Residents/patients in _____- term care facilities are one of the high-risk groups most likely to contract TB

Down

1. TB is transmitted when another person inhales a _____ of nuclei emitted by an infected person.

2. One of the signs and symptoms of TB is _____ sweats

3. It is important to teach a patient with TB to cover his or her mouth while _____

ANSWER KEY

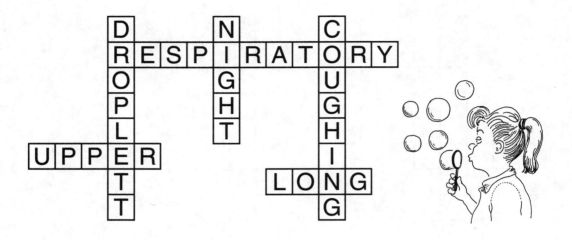

Across

4. respiratory
5. upper
6. long-

Down

1. droplet
2. night
3. coughing

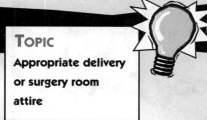
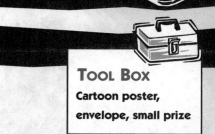
LABOR AND DELIVERY CARTOON CAPERS

Preparation

1. Make the ready-to-use Cartoon Capers page into a poster.

2. Copy the answer key for your own reference.

3. Hang the poster in the lounge or restroom area of your unit.

4. Attach an envelope to the bottom to collect entry forms.

Implementation

1. At the end of the week, collect the contents of the envelope and have a drawing from all the correct entries for a small token prize.

2. Post the correct answers the next week with the names of all those who gave the correct answers.

3. Continue to create cartoons by hand or clip art to reinforce important issues on the unit.

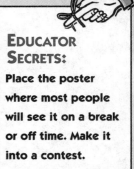

EDUCATOR
SECRETS:
Place the poster
where most people
will see it on a break
or off time. Make it
into a contest.

By: Michele Deck, MEd,
BSN, RN, ACCE-R

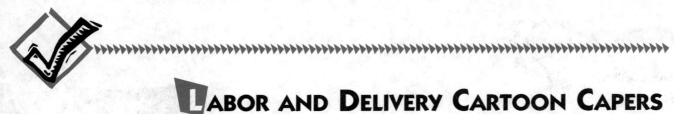

LABOR AND DELIVERY CARTOON CAPERS

Directions: Can you identify which four items this nurse is missing?

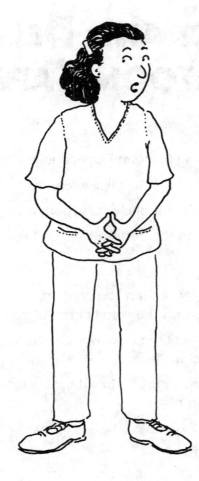

She is a nurse working labor and delivery today.
She is going into a delivery room any second.
What is she missing in her attire?

Here's a fun new way to review important information and win prizes at the same time! All you have to do is to write down your name and the answer to the above questions about delivery room attire, and you will be eligible for a prize drawing. Place your answers in the envelope provided below. Good luck!

LABOR AND DELIVERY CARTOON CAPERS

ANSWER KEY

Missing cap ———

Missing mask ———

Missing smile
(bonus answer!)

Missing gloves

Missing
shoe covers ———

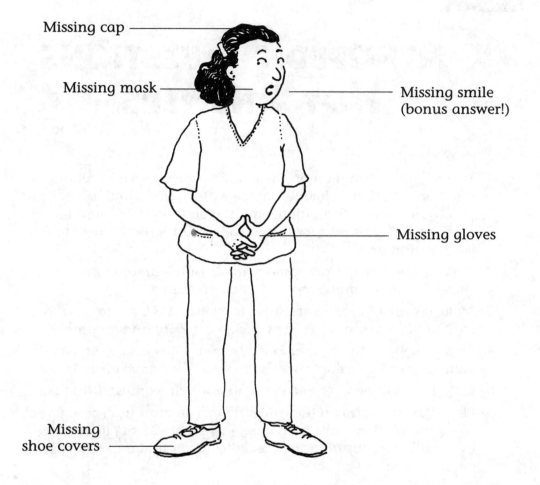

Answer: She is missing her hat, mask, gloves, and shoe covers.
(Bonus answer—a smile!)

20–30 minutes

TOPIC

Orthopedic information

TOOL BOX

Game board with categories and point amounts on overhead transparency (or poster), answer sheet, question sheet, buzzing device, Post-it™ notes, small prizes

ORTHOPEDIC QUESTIONS, NOT ANSWERS

Preparation

1. Review the information on the ready-to-use answers sheet and questions sheet. If it does not agree with your institution's policies, procedures, and information, edit it. (You'll need to adapt the answers and questions for the category "Orthopedic Docs" to fit your institution.)

2. Make an overhead transparency made of the amount and category sheet. (A poster can be made instead, if desired.)

3. Make a copy of the answer sheet for yourself. This is for you to read to the learners when they pick a category and an amount.

4. Make a copy of the answer key questions. This is for you to check your learners' question response to see if they are correct.

5. Obtain a buzzing device to determine which team rings in first.

6. Place Post-it™ notes on the category and amount transparency squares after they have been chosen. This blocks the light of the overhead projector from the ineligible boxes and makes it easier to see what can still be chosen.

7. Collect small prizes or goodies (fruit, Post-it™ notes, etc.) to award to the participants at the end of the activity.

Implementation

1. Divide the group into two or more teams of three to six learners.

2. Explain that the teams may collaborate on the questions.

3. Pick a team to go first. Display the playing board on the overhead projector. A spokesperson for the team selects a category and an amount.

continued

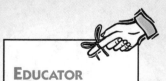

EDUCATOR SECRETS:

Set a fun atmosphere and equalize participation as much as possible.

By: Amanda Martin, MEd, BSN, RN, CNOR

ORTHOPEDIC QUESTIONS, NOT ANSWERS *continued*

4. The instructor reads the answer from that category and amount.

5. The team can discuss their ideas quietly for up to five seconds before answering.

6. A team representative states the question that fits the answer the instructor has given.

7. If the question given is correct, the team is awarded points based on how much their question was worth. If the answer is incorrect, the instructor can give the other team a chance to answer, or simply reveal the correct answer.

8. Points are tallied for each team.

9. After all answers are given, the team with the most points wins.

10. Prizes are awarded to all participants. Because their knowledge has increased, they are all winners.

ORTHOPEDIC QUESTIONS, NOT ANSWERS

AMOUNT AND CATEGORY SHEET

Directions: This playing board can be made into an overhead transparency or poster.

Potpourri	Standards and Protocols	Dem Bones	Orthopedic Docs	Traction
1	1	1	1	1
2	2	2	2	2
3	3	3	3	3
4	4	4	4	4
5	5	5	5	5

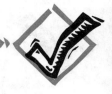

ORTHOPEDIC QUESTIONS, NOT ANSWERS

ANSWERS

Directions: This playing board can be made into an overhead transparency or poster.

Potpourri	Standards and Protocols	Dem Bones	Orthopedic Docs	Traction
Pain control device for *most* total joints	Absence of distal pulses; cool extremity; cyanotic nailbeds	Sling and swath used in this surgery	The "Hand" doctor	Types of traction that usually involve belts, halters, wraps, or boots
Must be changed at least every eight hours	Skin care, self care, safety	Requires replacement of acetabulum and femur head	Our newest staff physician	Type of traction sometimes placed pre-op for hip fractures
Never use powders or lotions around this type of incision	Call anesthesia; call physician	Patella	Goes by his middle name	Can only be applied by physician
Most common bone fractures by little old ladies	Must assess temp, WBC, drainage and dressing as indication of this	Small bone of lower leg	His total hip patients *always* travel by stretcher	Skin assessment; neurovascular checks; free hanging weights
Above the level of the heart	Responsible for patient's progress and activity post-op	Complication more common to long bone fractures	Wide receiver for the Denver Broncos—has Superbowl ring	Type of traction that can be used intermittently

169

ORTHOPEDIC QUESTIONS, NOT ANSWERS

ANSWER KEY QUESTIONS

Directions: This playing board can be made into an overhead transparency or poster.

Potpourri	Standards and Protocols	Dem Bones	Orthopedic Docs	Traction
What is a PCA pump?	What are the signs and symptoms of vascular impairment?	What is shoulder surgery?	Who is Dr. _____?	What is skin traction?
What is a hemovac?	What protocols are used most for ortho patients?	What is a total hip replacement?	Who is Dr. _____?	What is Buck's traction?
What is any ortho incision?	What to do for inadequate pain control?	What is the kneecap?	Who is Dr. _____?	What is skeletal traction?
What is the hip?	What is wound healing?	What is the fibula?	Who is Dr. _____?	What is the nursing care of the patient in traction?
How high do you elevate an extremity in a cast?	Who is physical therapy?	What is a fat embolus?	Who is Dr. _____?	What is pelvic traction (belt, not sling)?

Pain management focusing on PCA and epidural. This activity can also be used for other topics, including drugs and dosages, side effects, or any matching content.

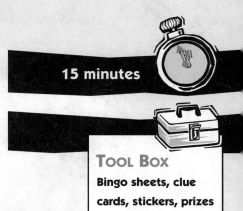

15 minutes

TOOL BOX

Bingo sheets, clue cards, stickers, prizes

CLUE BINGO

Preparation

1. Make a copy of the ready-to-use bingo sheet for each participant. Make a copy for yourself also.

2. Create clue cards, one card for each of the squares on the bingo sheet. The clues should be descriptions of the items in the squares.

3. Obtain some inexpensive, fun stickers. Each clue giver must have a number of these.

4. Collect some rewards for bingo winners.

Implementation

1. Divide the group into two parts with at least half (or six to eight people) in group A.

2. Group A are the clue givers and are given clue cards.

3. Group A members position themselves throughout the room.

4. Group B are the seekers and have bingo cards. They circulate among the clue givers.

5. Clue givers (A) have two to three clues on each card so they can be quizzed several times by the same person. The clue givers read the clues one at a time, waiting for an answer attempt after each clue from the individual seekers.

6. The faster the seeker (B) recognizes the answer on his or her bingo card, the more squares the seeker can quickly cover. When the correct answer is given, the clue givers (A) give stickers out to cover that square.

7. After two to three bingos are called out, the game stops.

8. As each bingo is called, provide a reward.

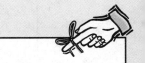

EDUCATOR SECRETS:

For a surprise twist, award all the learners a recognition prize for their efforts.

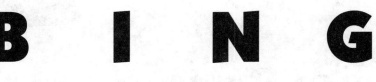

B	I	N	G	O
C 5	20%	Aspirin	CRNA	T 12
8	6–12 hrs	A 8	Morphine	Naloxone
T 1	Blood patch	**FREE**	T 6	Lipophilic
25%	T 4	Ephedrine	Ice	Marcaine
Alcohol	Yellow	Rostral	T 10	15

TOPIC
Pharmacology review.
This activity can be
adapted to any
content.

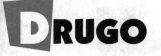

DRUGO

TOOL BOX
Drugo cards, clue
sheet, cupcakes or
small prizes for the
whole class, pens or
pencils

Preparation

1. Make a copy of the ready-to-use Drugo sheet for each participant.
2. Copy the Drugo clues sheet for your reference.
3. Obtain cupcakes or small prizes for the whole class.
4. Make sure each participant has a pen or pencil.

Implementation

1. Hand out the cards and tell the learners to cross off the appropriate item for each clue.
2. The first person to have five boxes crossed off in a row horizontally, vertically, or diagonally wins. He or she should shout out "Drugo!"
3. Students will get to the twentieth clue before calling "Drugo." The first nineteen positions of answers will not lead to a Drugo no matter what order they are in. The twentieth clue will give a Drugo no matter how the card is set up.

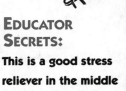

EDUCATOR SECRETS:
This is a good stress
reliever in the middle
of a pharmacology
review for a test.

By: Janet Fitts, BSN, RN,
CEN, EMT-P

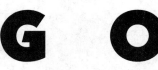

D R U G O

Normal saline	Tablet	Procardia	Calcium	Adenocard
Epinephrine 1:10,000	Meperidine	Lasix	ETOH	Atropine
Oxygen	Naloxone	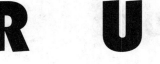	Beta	IV
Thrombo-lytics	Oxytocin	Capsule	Dextrose 50%	Nitrous oxide
IM	Proventil	Epinephrine 1:1,000	Alpha	Lidocaine

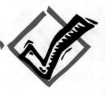

DRUGO

CLUES

1. I am the drug of choice in pulmonary edema.

2. I am the quickest and most dangerous route of administration.

3. I am the first drug of choice to all patients.

4. I am administered very rapidly for supraventricular tachycardia.

5. I am a synthetic narcotic, good for pain.

6. I am the first drug in anaphylactic shock.

7. You must find out if your patient has had a recent CVA before administering us.

8. I make mom stop bleeding heavily after the baby is born.

9. I am the receptor that increases the heart rate when stimulated.

10. I am given after a Verapamil overdose.

11. I am the drug route that goes deep into the gluteus.

12. I can be given for malathion poisoning.

13. I like to wake up a diabetic who had too much insulin.

14. I am often round and white, and I taste bitter.

15. I am a gas that is mixed and inhaled for pain relief from a mask.

16. I am the most frequently administered drug during a cardiac arrest.

17. I am inhaled to open the bronchioles and make it easier to breathe.

18. I am the receptor that causes peripheral vasoconstriction when stimulated.

19. I am the only capsule that is supposed to be punctured and squirted.

20. I am a liquid often consumed in larger amounts than reported.

21. I make patients breathe faster when they have over-dosed on narcotics.

22. I am an isotonic IV solution that is used in trauma.

23. I live in a gelatin casing and am more easily swallowed.

24. I am the first line drug to treat ventricular tachycardia with a pulse.

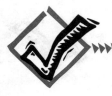

DRUGO

ANSWERS

1. I am the drug of choice in pulmonary edema. (*Lasix*)
2. I am the quickest and most dangerous route of administration. (*IV*)
3. I am the first drug of choice to all patients. (*Oxygen*)
4. I am administered very rapidly for supraventricular tachycardia. (*Adenocard*)
5. I am a synthetic narcotic, good for pain. (*Meperidine*)
6. I am the first drug in anaphylactic shock. (*Epi 1:1000*)
7. You must find out if your patient has had a recent CVA before administering us. (*Thrombolytics*)
8. I make mom stop bleeding heavily after the baby is born. (*Oxytocin*)
9. I am the receptor that increases the heart rate when stimulated. (*Beta*)
10. I am given after a Verapamil overdose. (*Calcium*)
11. I am the drug route that goes deep into the gluteus. (*IM*)
12. I can be given for malathion poisoning. (*Atropine*)
13. I like to wake up a diabetic who had too much insulin. (*Dextrose 50%*)
14. I am often round and white, and I taste bitter. (*Tablet*)
15. I am a gas that is mixed and inhaled for pain relief from a mask. (*Nitrous oxide*)
16. I am the most frequently administered drug during a cardiac arrest. (*Epi 1:10,000*)
17. I am inhaled to open the bronchioles and make it easier to breathe. (*Proventil*)
18. I am the receptor that causes peripheral vasoconstriction when stimulated. (*Alpha*)
19. I am the only capsule that is supposed to be punctured and squirted. (*Procardia*)
20. I am a liquid often consumed in larger amounts than reported. (*ETOH*)
21. I make patients breathe faster when they have overdosed on narcotics. (*Naloxone*)
22. I am an isotonic IV solution that is used in trauma. (*Normal saline*)
23. I live in a gelatin casing and am more easily swallowed. (*Capsule*)
24. I am the first line drug to treat ventricular tachycardia with a pulse. (*Lidocaine*)

TOPIC

Diagnostic tests.
This activity can be
adapted for use with
matching item
content of any kind.

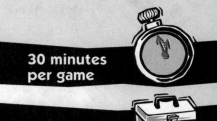

TOOL BOX

Game board, answer
key, small prizes
(optional)

DIAGNOSTIC DUOS

Preparation

*This activity matches diagnostic test names with a short description
of each.*

1. Create a poster board with a rebus puzzle on it.
2. Divide an identical size piece of poster paper into twenty-four
   rectangular board pieces.
3. On the rectangles, write the names of twelve tests and
   corresponding brief descriptions following the model Diagnostic
   Duos Game 1 and Game 2.
4. On the reverse side of the rectangles, number from one to twenty-
   four. (See Diagnostic Duos model.)
5. Place a *small* piece of velcro in the top middle of the rectangles
   front and back.
6. Place pieces of velcro throughout the picture background so that
   the rectangles can be attached in numerical order to cover the
   picture.

Implementation

1. Divide the group into two or more teams.
2. Each team chooses a spokesperson.
3. This person selects two numbers hoping the test and the description
   will match. If they do, they are removed from the board.
4. If they do not match, the next team takes a turn.
5. The teams continue to play until all the tests match.
6. Puzzle is solved by all teams writing down their guesses.
7. The winning team receives a small prize.

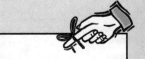

**EDUCATOR
SECRETS:**

Make the picture
puzzle difficult so
that all the matches
must be revealed
before the puzzle is
correctly guessed.

By: Michele Deck, MEd, BSN, RN, ACCE-R
Nancy Hennen, BSN, RNC

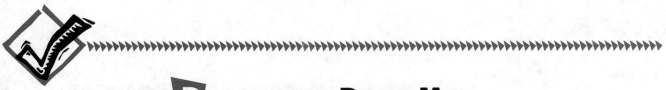

DIAGNOSTIC DUOS MODEL

Directions: This model can be made into an overhead transparency.

1	2	3	4
5	6	7	8
9	10	11	12
13	14	15	16
17	18	19	20
21	22	23	24

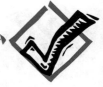

DIAGNOSTIC DUOS

GAME 1

Directions: This playing board can be made into an overhead transparency.

Thoracentesis/ paracentesis	EMG	Peripheral circulation	Blood vessels and the organs they supply
Insert needle between vertebra to withdraw spinal fluid	Proctoscopy	Endoscopy	Nuclear medicine
Electrical activity of the brain	Ultrasound	Electrical impulses of the muscles	EEG
Electrical activity of the beating heart	Withdraw fluid from around lungs and abdomen	DVI	Bouncing sound waves
Lumbar puncture	Vascular lab	Physiologic functions of the organs	ECG
Bronchoscopy	Exam of internal structures by inserting a lighted instrument into area	Endo of colon and rectum	Endo of trachea and bronchi

179

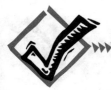

DIAGNOSTIC DUOS

GAME 1 ANSWER KEY

20	ECG	13	Electrical activity of the beating heart
12	EEG	9	Electrical activity of the brain
2	EMG	11	Electrical impulses of the muscles
10	Ultrasound	16	Bouncing sound waves
15	DVI	4	Blood vessels and the organs they supply
8	Nuclear medicine	19	Physiologic functions of the organs
18	Vascular lab	3	Peripheral circulation
1	Thoracentesis/ paracentesis	14	Withdraw fluid from around lungs and abdomen
7	Endoscopy	22	Exam of internal structures by inserting a lighted instrument into area
21	Bronchoscopy	24	Endo of trachea and bronchi
6	Proctoscopy	23	Endo of colon and rectum
17	Lumbar puncture	5	Insert needle between vertebra to withdraw spinal fluid

DIAGNOSTIC DUOS

GAME 2

Directions: This playing board can be made into an overhead transparency.

KUB	Lower intestines, digestive tract	Chest x-ray	Breast tissue
Blood vessels	MRI	IVP	Urinary tract
Magnetic internal anatomy	Esophagus, intestines, and small bowel	CAT scan	Angiogram
Kidney, ureter, and urinary bladder	Gall bladder and its ducts	Myelogram	Diary
Cross sections	Cholecystogram	Spinal canal	Lung, rib, and upper spine
Barium enema	Holter monitor	Mammogram	Upper GI

DIAGNOSTIC DUOS

GAME 2 ANSWER KEY

3 Chest x-ray		**20** Lung, rib, and upper spine	
1 KUB		**13** Kidney, ureter, and urinary bladder	
24 Upper GI		**10** Esophagus, stomach, and small bowel	
21 Barium enema		**2** Lower intestines, digestive tract	
18 Cholecystogram		**14** Gall bladder and its ducts	
12 Angiogram		**5** Blood vessels	
23 Mammogram		**4** Breast tissue	
6 MRI		**9** Magnetic internal anatomy	
11 CAT scan		**17** Cross sections	
22 Holter monitor		**16** Diary	
15 Myelogram		**19** Spinal canal	
7 IVP		**8** Urinary tract	

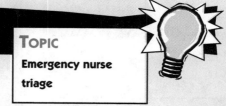
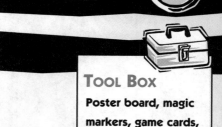

TOOL BOX
Poster board, magic markers, game cards, game rules

THE TRIAGE GAME

Preparation

1. Copy the Triage game board from the example. Or use it as a guide to develop your own board that shows the layout of your Emergency Department (ED). Make it as realistic as possible.

2. Cut game cards that are approximately 2" by 4" using two different colors.

3. On one color card write patient scenarios that are typical of the types of patients that you admit to your ED. You may include chief complaint, vital signs and symptoms, etc. These are the **patient cards**.

4. On the other color cards write individual events that may occur in your ED that may disrupt the normal patient flow. Examples are "Patient codes in Triage," "Six students arrive from a bus accident," or questions involving visiting policies, etc. These are the **event cards.**

5. Develop Triage game rules based on your ED's policies and procedures. The game rules should cover placement and handling of patients, movement of patients throughout the entire facility, and triage decisions based on various events. Your game rules should include your ED's policies and procedures.

6. Make a copy of the "games rules" for each participant.

Implementation

1. The game is played with one or more people. Each player or team of players should have one copy of the game board.

2. Each employee or team picks a patient card, then places it in the proper location on the game board. Patient placement depends on your ED's policies and procedures.

3. Use your "game rules" to move the patient(s) through the system. Triage patients according to your policies and procedures.

4. Event cards are introduced at intervals by the game leader. This adds excitement to the game and creates realistic events to the game.

5. This activity gives the learner(s) simulation experience and is valuable to new orientees prior to being placed in actual clinical situations.

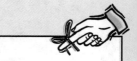

EDUCATOR SECRETS:
Be available to act as a resource for questions.

By: Susan Thornton, MEd, RN, CEN

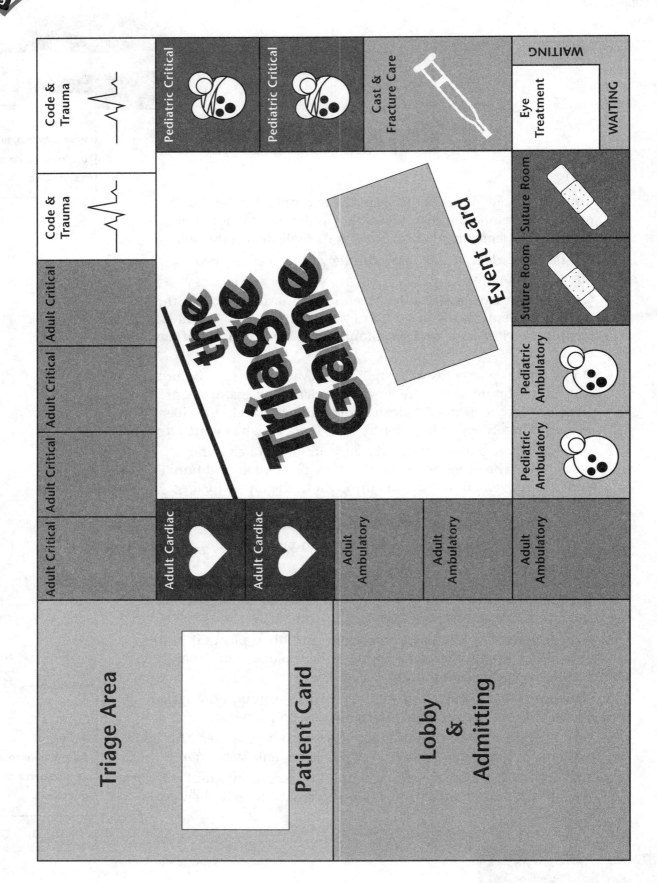

TOPIC

Lead placement for ECGs. This activity could be adapted to fit administration of other diagnostic equipment.

WHEEL OF PLACEMENT

TOOL BOX

Wheel of Placement; vowels with questions on back; skeleton or large picture of chest; V1, V2, V3, V4, V5, V6 placement circles; small pieces of candy, buzzers, ball

Preparation

1. Copy the ready-to-use Wheel of Placement.

2. Attach the small cardboard arrow to the center of the wheel using a pivot paper clip. This allows the arrow to spin.

3. Copy the Chest Lead Placement page or obtain a skeleton or large picture of the chest.

4. Copy the vowels and vowel selection questions back-to-back on the copy machine.

5. Cut the vowels/questions apart on the black lines.

6. Copy the placement circles, and cut them apart.

7. Set up a flipchart, chalkboard, or overhead with a mystery category word puzzle on it, such as *Lead Placement*. Leave a box or space visible for each letter in the puzzle.

8. Obtain some small pieces of candy.

Implementation

1. Divide the group into two or more teams (six to eight players is a good size).

2. Tell the group in which category the puzzle fits. For example, "It is a person."

3. Spin the arrow on the wheel. Be sure to spin and stop on all the areas. When it lands on an item, such as V3, the team that buzzes first controls the question.

continued

EDUCATOR SECRETS:

Play can continue with more puzzles until all areas of the wheel are covered.

By: Kathy Sciborski, MLT, (ASCP)

4. That team must tell where V3 goes (midway between V2 and V4), and they must come up to the skeleton or picture and place the V3 lead appropriately.

5. If they do this correctly, the team can pick a letter to solve the mystery category puzzle. If they want to buy a vowel, they must answer an extra question or do the activity on the back of the vowel they pick. If the team answers incorrectly, the other team gets to spin.

6. Play continues until a team solves the puzzle.

7. All of the teams receive prizes.

WHEEL OF PLACEMENT

SPINNER

Directions:

1. Cut out wheel.

2. Cut out arrow.

3. Paste arrow on cardboard.

4. Place arrow on wheel with a pivot paper clip.

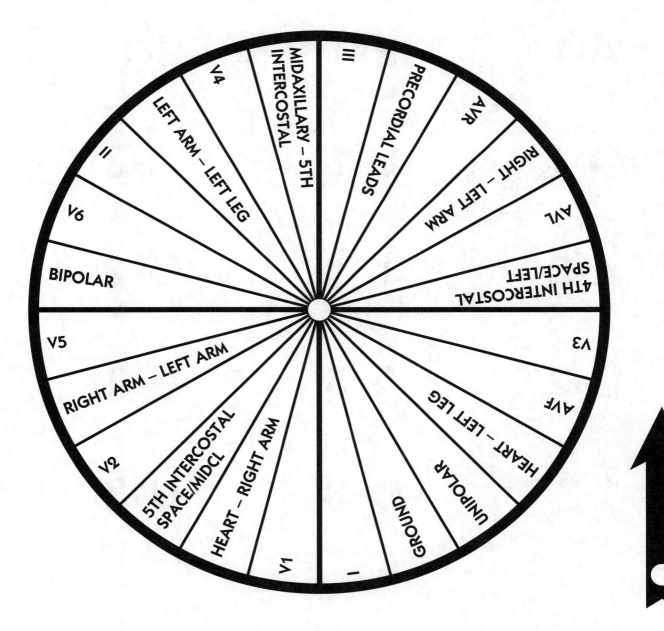

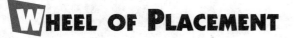

WHEEL OF PLACEMENT

VOWEL SELECTIONS

Directions:

1. Copy the Vowel Selections and Vowel Selection Questions (next page) back-to-back on the copy machine.

2. Cut out vowel/question cards.

A-1	E-1	I-1
O-1	U-1	A-2
E-2	I-2	O-2
U-2	A-3	E-3
I-3	O-3	U-3

WHEEL OF PLACEMENT

VOWEL SELECTION QUESTIONS

(These are just examples; you can make up your own)

Directions:

1. Copy the Vowel Selections and Vowel Selection Questions (preceding page) back-to-back on the copy machine.

2. Cut out vowel/question cards.

What's the first name of the vice president of the United States? **I-1**	How many employees work here? **E-1**	What's the only bird that gives leather? **A-1**
How many leads make up an ECG? **A-2**	Say, "Peter Piper picked a peck of pickled peppers" six times. **U-1**	Where can you find the organization's mission statement? **O-1**
When would you do a rhythm strip only? **O-2**	How many points are there on the Statue of Liberty's crown? **I-2**	Jump up and down on one foot while turning in a circle four times. **E-2**
Pat your head and rub your stomach for ten seconds. **E-3**	Who is our CEO? **A-3**	Sing the lyrics to "I'm a Little Teapot." **U-2**
How many employees make up the ECG department? **U-3**	Pass the ball to all members of your group without using any hands. **O-3**	In what state is John F. Kennedy buried? **I-3**

Answers: I-1—*Right now its Al;* **A-1**—*Ostrich;* **A-2**—*twelve;* **O-2**—*we don't anymore, must be done with chest leads;* **I-2**—*seven;* **I-3**—*Virginia*

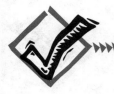

WHEEL OF PLACEMENT

CHEST LEAD PLACEMENT IDENTIFICATION CUTOUTS

Directions:

1. Cut out circles for placement on Skeleton or Chest Lead Placement Picture.

2. Use double-sided tape on the back of each circle so it will stick.

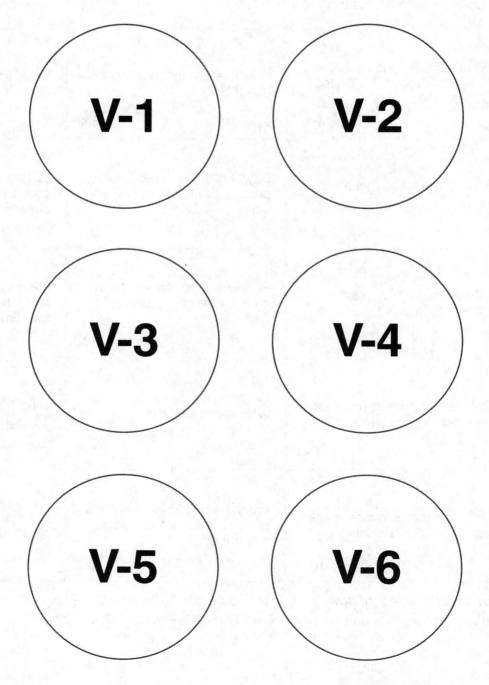

WHEEL OF PLACEMENT

CHEST LEAD PLACEMENT

Directions: Enlarge on poster paper or use as overhead.

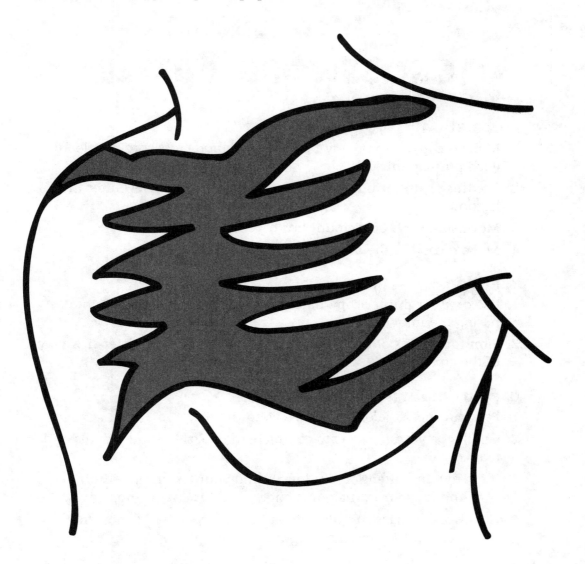

ANSWER KEY

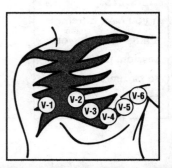

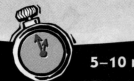

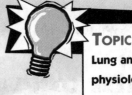

TOOL BOX
Lung Lingo crossword puzzle, pens or pencils, answer key

LUNG LINGO CROSSWORD PUZZLE

Preparation

1. Make a copy of the ready-to-use Lung Lingo crossword puzzle for each participant.
2. Use this as an introduction to the lesson or as a review after the lesson.
3. Make sure each participant has a pen or pencil.
4. Make a copy of the answer key.

Variation

1. Use a poster printer copy machine to turn the crossword into a poster-size image.
2. Plan for groups of two to six to discuss and fill in a poster-size copy of the crossword puzzle before or after your lesson.

Implementation

1. Pass out the large or small crossword puzzle.
2. Challenge your learners to complete the puzzle as individuals or as teams.
3. If energy and attention are low during your lesson presentation, stop and let your participants engage in this energizing activity.
4. Crossword puzzles can also be sent out days or weeks after the lesson as reinforcement of important concepts.

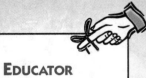

EDUCATOR SECRETS:
If you have different ability levels in your session, pair learners to maximize benefits to all.

By: Nancy Hennen, BSN, RNC

Lung Lingo Crossword Puzzle

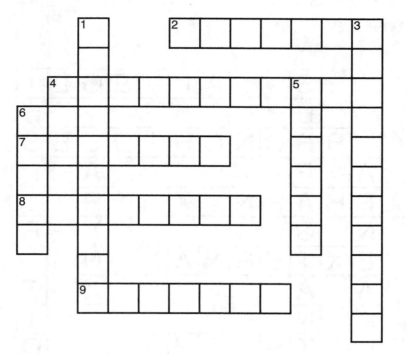

Across

2. Clusters of air sacs
4. The smallest subdivisions of the bronchi
7. Another name for the throat
8. Gas exchange between blood and alveoli
9. The windpipe

Down

1. The alveoli produce _____
3. This is the ACTIVE phase of breathing
5. The voice box
6. The temporary cessation of breathing

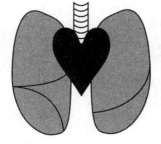

Lung Lingo Crossword Puzzle

Answer Key

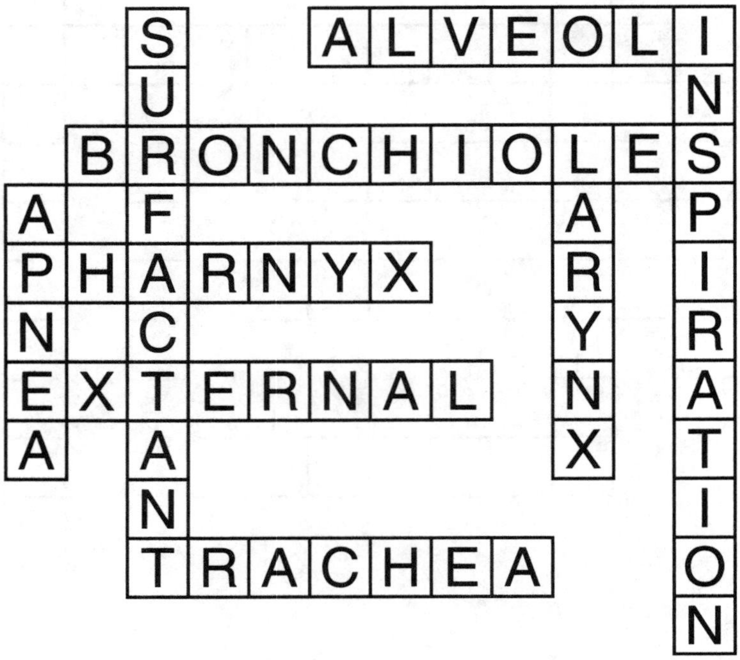

Across

2. alveoli
4. bronchioles
7. pharynx
8. external (respiration)
9. trachea

Down

1. surfactant
3. inspiration
5. larynx
6. apnea

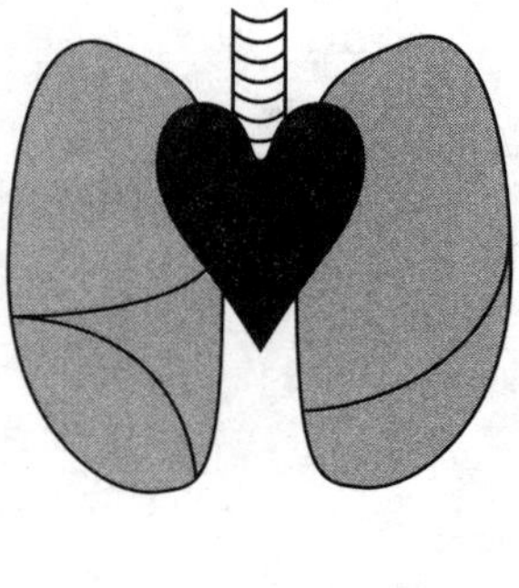

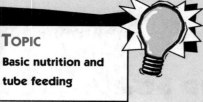
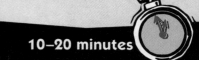
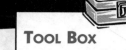

TOOL BOX
Nutritional Nonsense
fill-in-the-blank
sheets, word search
sheets, pens or
pencils, answer key

NUTRITIONAL NONSENSE

Preparation

1. Make a copy of the ready-to-use Nutritional Nonsense word search and fill-in-the-blanks sheets for each participant.

2. Make a copy the answer key.

3. Use this puzzle as an introduction to the lesson or as a review after the lesson.

4. Make sure each participant has a pen or pencil.

Variation

1. Use a poster printer copy machine to turn the word search puzzle into a poster-size image.

2. Plan for groups of two to six to discuss and fill in a poster-size copy of the word search puzzle before or after your lesson.

Implementation

1. Distribute the Nutritional Nonsense fill-in-the-blank sheets and the large or small word search puzzle.

2. Challenge your learners to complete the word search puzzle as individuals or as teams.

3. Invite the participants to find the answers to the blanks in the word search puzzle. The words may appear vertically, horizontally, diagonally, or backward.

4. If energy and attention are low during your lesson presentation, stop and let your participants engage in this energizing activity.

5. Word search puzzles can also be sent out days or weeks after the lesson as reinforcement of important concepts.

6. This serves as a fun and quick review and reinforcement of the content.

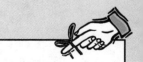

EDUCATOR SECRETS:
Challenge the
learners to fill in the
blanks first or race
against each team.

By: Nancy Hennen, BSN, RNC

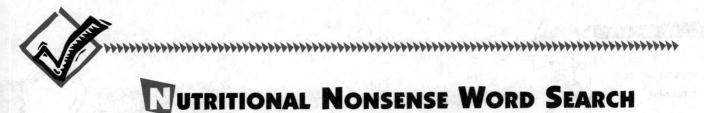

NUTRITIONAL NONSENSE WORD SEARCH

Directions: The answers to the questions on the Nutritional Nonsense fill-in-the-blanks sheet are hidden in the puzzle below. Words may be horizontal, vertical, or diagonal, and forward or backward. Circle the hidden words. Have fun!

```
C C Q P R G B K I J
E A Z G H M Z L V W
K L S N E S D I E N
P O L V D T T M I Q
D R A Q E A B F N L
J I R V M F J C K C
F E E I A Z X A S T
S S N I E T O R P O
T S I C O V X B T T
P T M P T N U O C S
P O X V F I S H W B
N M E N E R G Y O D
B A B C D E F D H H
D C G S T I U R F K
I H J K L M N A L N
R Q S S A C D T U V
K J H U P S Y E I J
W Y Z L L Q R S D E
C B L O M F N Z R S
L K P B T T P E G N
```

NUTRITIONAL NONSENSE
FILL-IN-THE-BLANKS

Directions: Listed below are statements concerning basic nutrition and tube feedings. The answers to the questions are hidden in the word search puzzle attached. The words may be horizontal, vertical, or diagonal, and forward or backward. Circle the hidden words in the puzzle. Have fun!

1. One of the four basic food groups is _____ and dairy products.

2. _____ provide energy.

3. _____ are important in bowel elimination.

4. These nutrients have specific functions, and the body cannot produce them. They are _____ .

5. _____ are important for bones, tooth, nerve, and muscle functions.

6. _____ and vegetables are a food group.

7. Meat and _____ are a food group.

8. When you record the fractions of food and fluid consumed, it is called a calorie _____ .

9. These nutrients are essential for tissue growth: _____ .

10. Too much fluid in the body can result in _____ .

11. Hyperalimentation is adequate nutrition given into the _____ and includes carbohydrates, proteins, and fats.

12. Tube feedings are given through a tube into the _____ .

13. It is essential to have 1500 ccs of _____ every day.

14. Fats provide twice the amount of _____ .

15. A gastrostomy tube is commonly called a _____ tube.

16. To prevent a gastrostomy tube from clogging, you should _____ it with 30 ccs of water after each feeding or aspiration.

17. An intermittent tube feeding may be called a _____ feeding.

NUTRITIONAL NONSENSE WORD SEARCH

Answers

1. milk
2. fats
3. carbohydrates
4. vitamins
5. minerals
6. fruits
7. fish
8. count
9. proteins
10. edema
11. vein
12. stomach
13. fluid
14. energy
15. PEG
16. flush
17. bolus

ANSWER KEY

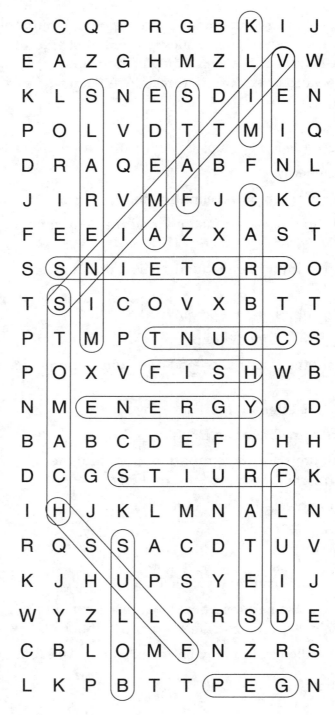

C C Q P R G B K I J
E A Z G H M Z L V W
K L S N E S D I E N
P O L V D T T M I Q
D R A Q E A B F N L
J I R V M F J C K C
F E E I A Z X A S T
S S N I E T O R P O
T S I C O V X B T T
P T M P T N U O C S
P O X V F I S H W B
N M E N E R G Y O D
B A B C D E F D H H
D C G S T I U R F K
I H J K L M N A L N
R Q S S A C D T U V
K J H U P S Y E I J
W Y Z L L Q R S D E
C B L O M F N Z R S
L K P B T T P E G N

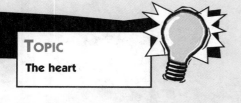
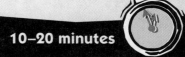
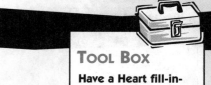
HAVE A HEART

Preparation

1. Make a copy of the ready-to-use Have a Heart fill-in-the-blank sheet for each participant.
2. Use this as an introduction to the lesson or as a review after the lesson.
3. Make sure each participant has a pen or pencil.
4. Make a copy of the answer key.

Variation

1. Use a poster printer copy machine to turn the sheet puzzle into a poster-size image.
2. Plan for groups of two to six to discuss and fill in a poster-size copy of the sheet before or after your lesson.

Implementation

1. Pass out Have a Heart fill-in-the-blank sheets.
2. Challenge your learners to complete the page as individuals or as teams.
3. If energy and attention are low during your lesson presentation, stop and let your participants engage in this energizing activity.
4. Fill-in-the-blank sheets can also be sent out days or weeks after the lesson as reinforcement of important concepts.

EDUCATOR SECRETS:
If you have different experience levels in your session, pair learners to maximize benefits to all.

HAVE A HEART

1. The ❤ serves as a _____ when it contracts and relaxes. It moves the _____ throughout the body.

2. The ❤ has two complete parts (halves), sometimes called the _____ ❤ and the _____ ❤.

3. Each half of the ❤ is divided into two chambers. The top chambers are called _____ and the bottom chambers are called _____.

4. The human ❤ beats about _____ times a minute.

5. The _____ carry blood TO the ❤.

6. The _____ carry blood FROM the ❤.

7. The ❤ is divided down the middle by the _____.

8. Blood is supplied to the ❤ by the right and left _____.

9. The right side of the ❤ pumps blood to the _____.

10. The left side of the ❤ pumps blood to the _____.

Have A Heart

Answer Key

1. The ❤ serves as a _____pump_____ when it contracts and relaxes. It moves the _____blood_____ throughout the body.

2. The ❤ has two complete parts (halves), sometimes called the _____left_____ ❤ and the _____right_____ ❤.

3. Each half of the ❤ is divided into two chambers. The top chambers are called _____atria_____ and the bottom chambers are called _____ventricles_____.

4. The human ❤ beats about _____60–100_____ times a minute.

5. The _____veins_____ carry blood TO the ❤.

6. The _____arteries_____ carry blood FROM the ❤.

7. The ❤ is divided down the middle by the _____septum_____.

8. Blood is supplied to the ❤ by the right and left _coronary arteries_.

9. The right side of the ❤ pumps blood to the _____body_____.

10. The left side of the ❤ pumps blood to the _____lungs_____.

TOOL BOX

Game board showing categories and point amounts on overhead transparency (or poster), answers sheet, questions sheet, a buzzing device, Post-it™ notes, small prizes

TOPIC

Handwashing, pulse, respiration and blood pressure, side rails, heating pads, douching, intake and output, gloving, catheter, dressing change, stool collection, 24-hour urine collection

PATIENT CARE QUESTIONS, NOT ANSWERS

Preparation

1. Review the information on the ready-to-use answers sheet and questions sheet. If it does not agree with your institution's policies, procedures, and information, edit it.

2. Have an overhead transparency made from the amount and category sheet. (A poster can be made instead if desired.)

3. Copy the answers sheet. This is for you to read to the learners when they pick a category and amount.

4. Copy the answer key questions. This is for you to check your learners' question responses to see if they are correct.

5. Obtain a buzzing device to determine which team rings in first.

6. Place Post-it™ notes on the category and amount transparency squares after they have been chosen. This blocks the light of the overhead projector from the ineligible boxes and makes it easier to see what can still be chosen.

7. Collect small prizes or goodies (fruit, Post-it™ notes, etc.) to award to the participants at the end of the activity.

Implementation

1. Divide the group into two or more teams of three to six learners.

2. Explain that the teams may collaborate on the questions.

continued

EDUCATOR SECRETS:

Equalize the competition if possible. Learners find it more fun and less stressful when everyone has a turn to answer.

By: Michele Deck, MEd, BSN, RN, ACCE-R
Nancy Hennen, BSN, RNC

PATIENT CARE QUESTIONS, NOT ANSWERS *continued*

3. Pick a team to go first. Display the playing board on the overhead projector. A spokesperson for the team selects a category and an amount.

4. The instructor reads the answer from that category and amount.

5. The teams can discuss their ideas quietly for up to five seconds before answering.

6. A team representative states the question that fits the answer the instructor has given.

7. If the question given is correct, the team is awarded points based on how much their question is worth. If the answer is incorrect, the other team can answer or the instructor can choose to reveal the answer.

8. Points are tallied for each team.

9. After all answers are given, the team with the most points wins.

10. Prizes are awarded to all participants. Because their knowledge has increased, they are all winners.

Patient Care Questions, Not Answers

Game 1 Amount and Category Sheet

Directions: This playing board can be made into an overhead transparency.

Scale-ing Down	On the Go	Jug-ling	Hot & Heavy	Heart Throb	Stop & Go	Spray & Wash
1	1	1	1	1	1	1
2	2	2	2	2	2	2
3	3	3	3	3	3	3
4	4	4	4	4	4	4
5	5	5	5	5	5	5

PATIENT CARE QUESTIONS, NOT ANSWERS

GAME 1 ANSWERS

Directions: This playing board can be made into an overhead transparency.

Spray & Wash	Stop & Go	Heart Throb	Hot & Heavy	Jug-ling	On the Go	Scale-ing Down
This is the easiest and most important way to prevent the spread of infection	It is the introduction of fluid into the rectum or lower colon to remove fecal material	You need this equipment to obtain a radial pulse	This type of heat penetrates better than dry heat	This is the name given to all urine collected for a full day	Stool specimens are collected to find this out	This is used to get an accurate weight on a patient who is unable to stand
Handwashing should be done at these times	These three factors influence bowel regularity	60 to 100	You observe for these three things during or after the application of a heating pad	You should discard this specimen	This should not be mixed with a stool specimen	You must never do this to a patient on a bed scale
These must stay lower than the elbows at all times when handwashing	The patient is placed in this position during an enema	The part of your hand that should never be used to take a radial pulse	The heating pad will not work if the chamber is not filled with this	The urine jug must be kept in this	The term OB on a stool slip stands for this	You must do this after you use the scale and it is returned to its storage area
You should use only these two items for washing your hands	The patient should hold an enema for this amount of time	You count the radial pulse for this period of time and multiply the rate by two	This happens to the heating pad if the connections are not hooked together tightly	You must have the patient do this before he or she leaves the floor for any reason	The term OCP is marked on a stool slip to check for this	You have to make sure that the frame is not doing this when you are measuring a patient's weight
This prevents your hands from chapping	The amount of water used in a cleansing enema	You listen with a stethoscope over this part of the heart to take an apical pulse	Have the patient report these signs to you if they occur while using the heating pad	You must rinse the bedpan, urinal, and graduated pitcher with this between voiding	You should place a stool specimen jar in this with the slip outside of it before it is sent to the lab	The patient is raised this far off the bed when using a bed scale to weigh him or her

PATIENT CARE QUESTIONS, NOT ANSWERS

GAME 1 ANSWER KEY QUESTIONS

Directions: This playing board can be made into an overhead transparency.

Scale-ing Down	What is a bed scale?	What is leave them alone?	What is plug it in?	What is touching anything?	What is one to three inches?
On the Go	What is blood, fat, or organisms?	What is urine, barium, enema solution, or suppositories?	What is occult blood?	What are parasites?	What is a plastic bag?
Jug-ling	What is a 24-hour urine collection?	What is the first voided specimen?	What is ice?	What is void?	What is sterile water?
Hot & Heavy	What is moist heat?	What is swelling, redness, or blisters?	What is distilled water?	What is water leaking from the port?	What is pain and decreased sensation?
Heart Throb	What is a watch with a second hand?	What is a normal adult pulse?	What is your thumb?	What is thirty seconds?	What is the apex?
Stop & Go	What is an enema?	What are diet, fluids, and privacy?	What is left side lying?	What is five minutes?	What is 1000 ccs?
Spray & Wash	What is handwashing?	What is before and after every patient contact?	What are the hands?	What is soap and water?	What is drying thoroughly?

PATIENT CARE QUESTIONS, NOT ANSWERS

GAME 2 AMOUNT AND CATEGORY SHEET

Directions: This playing board can be made into an overhead transparency.

Play Pen Safety	Up the Tubes	Touch Me Not	April Showers	Full of Hot Air	4 x 4 Fashion	Take Out
1	1	1	1	1	1	1
2	2	2	2	2	2	2
3	3	3	3	3	3	3
4	4	4	4	4	4	4
5	5	5	5	5	5	5

GAME 2 ANSWERS

Directions: This playing board can be made into an overhead transparency.

Take Out	4 x 4 Fashion	Full of Hot Air	April Showers	Touch Me Not	Up the Tubes	Play Pen Safety
The initials I and O stand for this	You need to pour this on a 4 x 4 to apply a wet to dry dressing	The rate is between twelve and twenty	It is the introduction of fluid into the vagina to cleanse or disinfect	These are used when an aseptic technique is performed, such as catheterization	This is the insertion of a sterile tube into the bladder	You never leave these down after patient care
Intake and output evaluate these two things	The transparent film dressing should be this much larger than the size of the wound	You should take respirations before or after you do this	The usual solution used for douching; some people are allergic to it	This is the part of the glove packaging that you can touch and still have the package remain sterile	You use this sort of motion to cleanse the meatus	This should be kept at the lowest position at all times
I and O are measured in this unit of measurement	This dressing is applied to the wound in a rolling motion and held for thirty seconds	It is important to see this rise and fall while taking respirations	The amount of fluid used to give a douche	You must keep your hands at this level of your body once your sterile gloves are on	You should leave the catheter in the bladder until this happens	Confused, sedated, or unconscious patients should have these up
The pitcher should be placed on this to measure the fluid	You should never do this when you are drying the area around a wound	This can change the rate of respirations	It is of utmost importance to provide this to the patient while you are giving a douche	You adjust your gloves only at this time	What you should instruct the patient to do as you insert the catheter	These should be placed in the locked position when transporting patients to and from them
You must instruct the patient and his or her family that these should be added to the I and O record	Once skin prep is applied, you need to let this happen	You count the respirations for this long and multiply by two	The patient is positioned like this before the douche	If you are right-handed, this is the glove you put on first	This side of the underpad faces the bed, not the patient	This piece of equipment must always be in reach of the patient in bed

PATIENT CARE QUESTIONS, NOT ANSWERS

GAME 2 ANSWER KEY QUESTIONS

Directions: This playing board can be made into an overhead transparency.

Take Out	4 x 4 Fashion	Full of Hot Air	April Showers	Touch Me Not	Up the Tubes	Play Pen Safety
What are intake and output?	What is saline?	What is the rate of normal adult respirations?	What is douching or vaginal irrigation?	What are sterile gloves?	What is catheterization?	What are side rails?
What are fluid balance and kidney function?	What is two inches?	What is taking a radial pulse?	What is Betadine?	What are the outside edges?	What is circular motion?	What is the bed?
What is ccs or mls?	What is a wafer dressing?	What is the patient's chest?	What is 1000 ccs?	What is the chest level?	What is when the bladder is completely drained?	What are side rails?
What is a level surface?	What is touch the wound?	What are activities, emotions, or some medications?	What is privacy?	What is when both gloves are on?	What is to take a deep breath?	What are wheelchairs, beds, or stretchers?
What are semisolids such as custard, ice cream, and jello?	What is let it dry?	What is thirty seconds?	What is flat on her back with knees bent and legs open?	What is the right glove?	What is the plastic side?	What is the call bell?

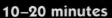
10–20 minutes

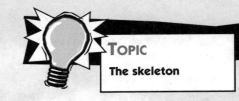

TOOL BOX

Name That Bone fill-in-the-blank sheet, pens or pencils, answer key

NAME THAT BONE!

Preparation

1. Make a copy of the ready-to-use Name That Bone fill-in-the-blank sheet for each participant.

2. Use this as an introduction to the lesson or as a review after the lesson.

3. Make sure each participant has a pen or pencil.

4. Make a copy of the answer key.

Variation

1. Use a poster printer copy machine to turn the sheet puzzle into a poster-size image.

2. Plan for groups of two to six to discuss and fill in a poster-size copy of the sheet before or after your lesson.

Implementation

1. Pass out the Name That Bone fill-in-the-blank sheets.

2. Challenge your learners to complete the page as individuals or as teams.

3. If energy and attention are low during your lesson presentation, stop and let your participants engage in this energizing activity.

4. Fill-in-the-blank sheets can also be sent out days or weeks after the lesson as reinforcement of important concepts.

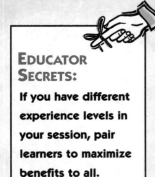

EDUCATOR SECRETS:

If you have different experience levels in your session, pair learners to maximize benefits to all.

By: Nancy Hennen, BSN, RNC

NAME THAT BONE

Directions: Match the name of the following bones to the letters on the picture of the skeleton. Place the correct letter in the blank beside the name of each bone.

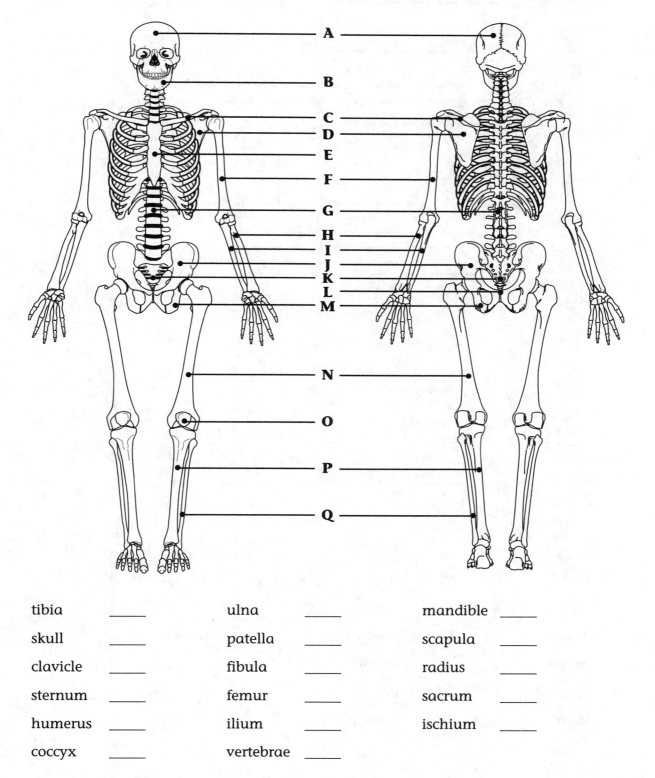

tibia	_____	ulna	_____	mandible	_____
skull	_____	patella	_____	scapula	_____
clavicle	_____	fibula	_____	radius	_____
sternum	_____	femur	_____	sacrum	_____
humerus	_____	ilium	_____	ischium	_____
coccyx	_____	vertebrae	_____		

211

NAME THAT BONE

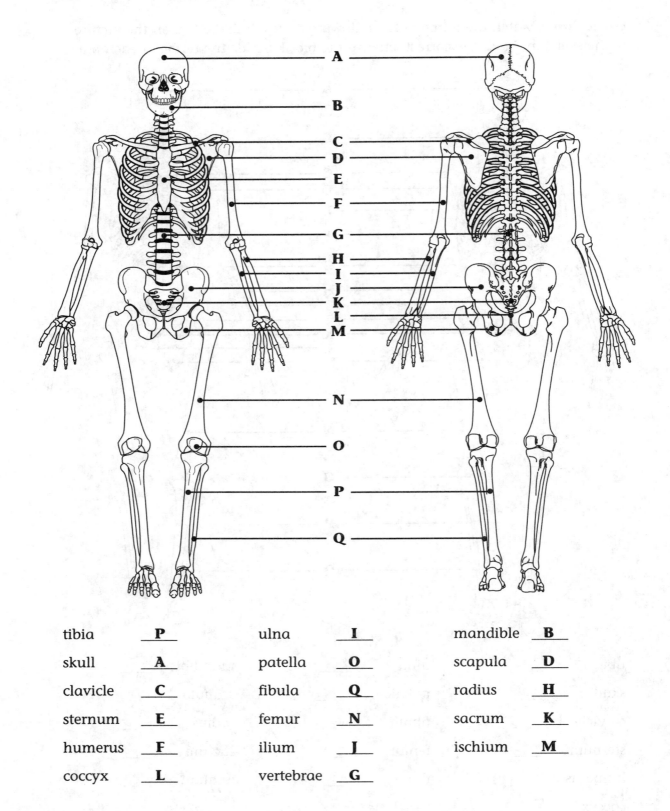

tibia	**P**	ulna	**I**	mandible	**B**
skull	**A**	patella	**O**	scapula	**D**
clavicle	**C**	fibula	**Q**	radius	**H**
sternum	**E**	femur	**N**	sacrum	**K**
humerus	**F**	ilium	**J**	ischium	**M**
coccyx	**L**	vertebrae	**G**		

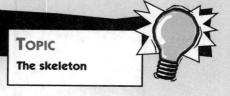

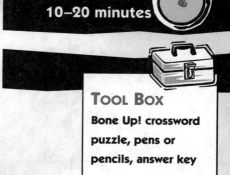

TOOL BOX
Bone Up! crossword puzzle, pens or pencils, answer key

BONE UP! CROSSWORD PUZZLE

Preparation

1. Make a copy of the ready-to-use Bone Up! crossword puzzle for each participant.

2. Use this as an introduction to the lesson or as a review after the lesson.

3. Make sure each participant has a pen or pencil.

4. Make a copy of the answer key.

Variation

1. Use a poster printer copy machine to turn the crossword into a poster-size image.

2. Plan for groups of two to six to discuss and fill in a poster-size copy of the crossword puzzle before or after your lesson.

Implementation

1. Pass out the large or small crossword puzzle.

2. Challenge your learners to complete the puzzle as individuals or as teams.

3. If energy and attention are low during your lesson presentation, stop and let your participants engage in this energizing activity.

4. Crossword puzzles can also be sent out days or weeks after the lesson as reinforcement of important concepts.

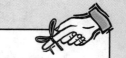

EDUCATOR SECRETS:
If you have different experience levels in your session, pair learners to maximize benefits to all.

By: Nancy Hennen, BSN, RNC

BONE UP! CROSSWORD PUZZLE

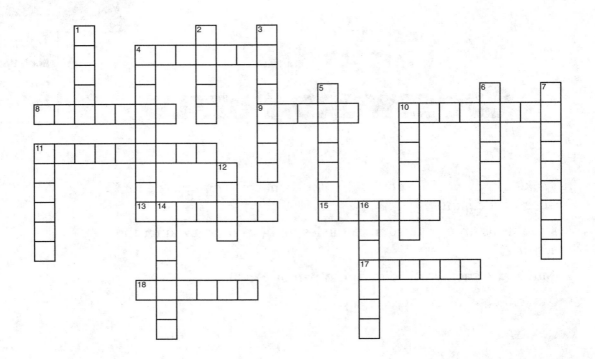

Across

4. This is your kneecap
8. This is your shoulder blade
9. This is the flared part of your hip bone (The skeleton is resting its hand there)
10. This is your collar bone
11. This is your heel
13. This is your breast bone
15. Your tailbone is connected to this bone (fusion of five bones)
17. Elvis shakes his
18. The larger of your forearm bones (thumb side)

Down

1. This is your shin bone
2. This is your thigh bone
3. This is your lower jaw bone
4. These are your fingers and toes
5. This is your upper arm bone
6. This is your calf bone
7. This is your spinal column
10. This bone protects your brain
11. This is your tailbone
12. The smaller bone in your forearm (little finger side)
14. These are your ankle bones
16. These are your wrist bones

Bone Up! Crossword Puzzle

Answer Key

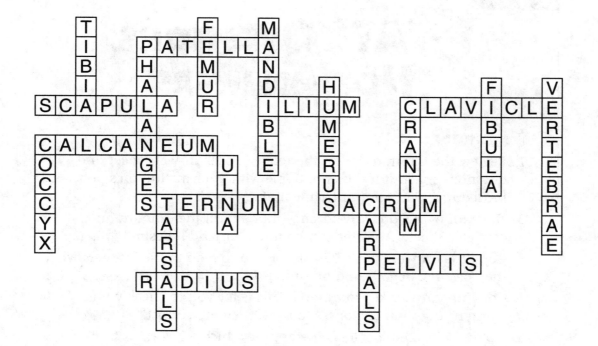

Across

4. patella
8. scapula
9. ilium
10. clavicle
11. calcaneum
13. sternum
15. sacrum
17. pelvis
18. radius

Down

1. tibia
2. femur
3. mandible
4. phalanges
5. humerus
6. fibula
7. vertebrae
10. cranium
11. coccyx
12. ulna
14. tarsals
16. carpals

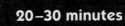
TOOL BOX

Game board with categories and point amounts on overhead transparency (or poster), answers sheet, questions sheet, buzzing device, Post-it™ notes, small prizes

STAT! QUESTIONS, NOT ANSWERS

Preparation

1. Review the information on the ready-to-use answers sheet and questions sheet. If it does not agree with your institution's policies, procedures, and information, edit it.

2. Have an overhead transparency made from the amount and category sheet. (A poster can be made instead if desired.)

3. Copy the answers sheet. This is for you to read to the learners when they pick a category and an amount.

4. Copy the answer key questions. This is for you to check your learners' question responses to see if they are correct.

5. Obtain a buzzing device to determine which team rings in first.

6. Place Post-it™ notes on the category and amount transparency squares after they have been chosen. This blocks the light of the overhead projector from the ineligible boxes and makes it easier to see what can still be chosen.

Implementation

1. Divide the group into two or more teams of three to six learners.

2. Explain that the teams may collaborate on the questions.

3. Pick a team to go first. Display the playing board on the overhead projector. A spokesperson for the team selects a category and an amount.

4. The instructor reads the answer from that category and amount.

5. The teams can discuss their ideas quietly for up to five seconds before answering.

continued

EDUCATOR SECRETS:

Set a fun atmosphere and equalize participation as much as possible.

By: Regina Lawless Phelps, MN, RN

STAT! QUESTIONS, NOT ANSWERS *continued*

6. A team representative states the question that fits the answer the instructor has given.

7. If the question given is correct, the team is awarded points based on how much their question was worth. If the answer is incorrect, the other team can answer or the instructor can choose to reveal the answer.

8. Points are tallied for each team.

9. After all answers are given, the team with the most points wins.

10. Prizes are awarded to all participants. Since their knowledge has increased, they are all winners.

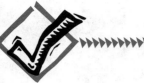

STAT! QUESTIONS, NOT ANSWERS

AMOUNT AND CATEGORY SHEET

Directions: This playing board can be made into an overhead transparency or poster.

Red River Valley	One Flew Over the Cuckoo's Nest	Gone with the Wind	Potpourri
100	100	100	100
200	200	200	200
300	300	300	300
400	400	400	400
500	500	500	500

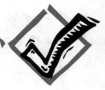

STAT! QUESTIONS, NOT ANSWERS

ANSWERS

Directions: This playing board can be made into an overhead transparency or poster.

Red River Valley	One Flew Over the Cuckoo's Nest	Gone with the Wind	Potpourri
The most common cause of noncardiac chest pain	Three factors indicating high risk for suicide	The presence of stridor, wheezing, and gasping respirations indicate this	An inherited condition triggered by administration of anesthesia
This nonlethal rhythm is a negative prognostic indicator of acute MI	A suicide attempter who took great pains to avoid discovery	The most common emergent event in the hospitalized adult	Three of the five types of drugs used to treat anaphylaxis
Preservation of heart muscle	Three causes of coma in adults	Dyspnea, tachycardia, tachypnea, and pain	Two types of shock that may show early rise of blood pressure
Three signs of coronary reperfusion	A Glasgow coma scale of 4 indicates this	S3	Tissue necrosis factor is now treated with this class of drugs
This is characteristic of papillary muscle rupture in acute MI	Three ways to decrease ICP	The sudden disappearance of wheezing in the asthmatic	Two causes of hypothermia in hospitalized patients

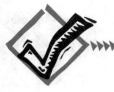

STAT! QUESTIONS, NOT ANSWERS

ANSWER KEY QUESTIONS

Directions: This playing board can be made into an overhead transparency or poster.

Red River Valley	One Flew Over the Cuckoo's Nest	Gone with the Wind	Potpourri
What is gastric pain?	What are male, adolescent, or greater than 45?	What is airway obstruction, partial?	What is malignant hyperthermia?
What is atrial fibrillation?	What is a lethal attempter?	What is pulmonary embolus?	What are adrenaline, antihistamines, xanthines, anticholinergics, steroids?
What is the primary goal in managing MI?	What are DM, CVA, trauma, OD, tumor?	What are the most common symptoms of a PE?	What are sepsis and neurogenic?
What are decreased pain, normal ST segment, and dysrhythmias?	What is a decreased neuro status?	What is often the first sign of impending heart failure?	What are murine monoclonal antibodies?
What is a loud, holosystolic murmur?	What is raise HOB, decrease CO_2, steroids, decrease fluids, diuretics, barbiturate coma?	What is the third stage of asthma?	What are rapid infusion of cold fluids and induced barbituates?

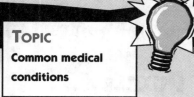
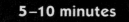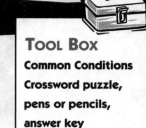
COMMON CONDITIONS CROSSWORD PUZZLE

Preparation

1. Make a copy of the ready-to-use Common Conditions crossword puzzle for each participant.
2. Use this as an introduction to the lesson or as a review after the lesson.
3. Make sure each participant has a pen or pencil.
4. Make a copy of the answer key.

Variation

1. Use a poster printer copy machine to turn the crossword into a poster-size image.
2. Plan for groups of two to six to discuss and fill in a poster-size copy of the crossword puzzle before or after your lesson.

Implementation

1. Pass out the large or small crossword puzzle.
2. Challenge your learners to complete the puzzle as individuals or as teams.
3. If energy and attention are low during your lesson presentation, stop and let your participants engage in this energizing activity.
4. Crossword puzzles can also be sent out days or weeks after the lesson as reinforcement of important concepts.

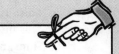

EDUCATOR SECRETS:
If you have different experience levels in your session, pair learners to maximize benefits to all.

By: Nancy Hennen, BSN, RNC
Linda Rodriguez

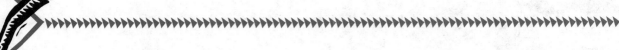

Common Conditions Crossword Puzzle

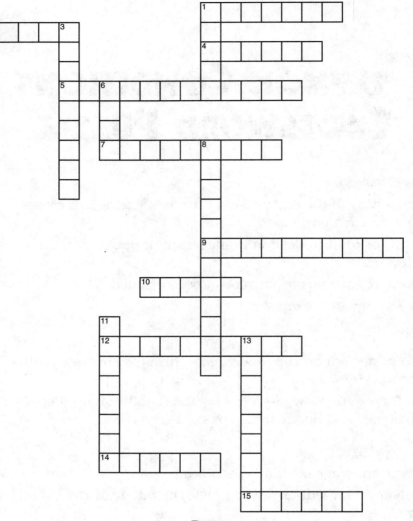

Across

1. Chronic bronchitis is an inflammation of the _____
2. This is due to a decreased blood flow to a part of the heart
4. This is a disease where air passages narrow
5. This disease is caused by narrowing of blood vessels
7. This disease is an inflammation of lung tissue
9. Signs and symptoms of this disease include a mask-like facial expression and tremors
10. In coronary artery disease, the arteries around this organ become narrow
12. This disease causes gradual memory loss (especially recent events), and personality and behavior changes
14. A CVA occurs when the blood supply is interrupted to a part of the brain. What is the common term for a CVA?
15. A lack of blood to the heart causes tissue death in the heart. This is commonly called a heart _____

Down

1. Chronic Brain Syndrome is a disease in which changes occur in the cells of the _____
3. What disease is joint inflammation?
6. In congestive heart failure the heart is unable to normally_____
8. A bone disorder in which bones become porous and brittle
11. In diabetes mellitus this organ fails to secrete an adequate amount of insulin
13. This is a disease in which the alveolar become enlarged and less elastic

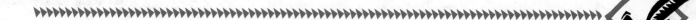

COMMON CONDITIONS CROSSWORD PUZZLE

ANSWER KEY

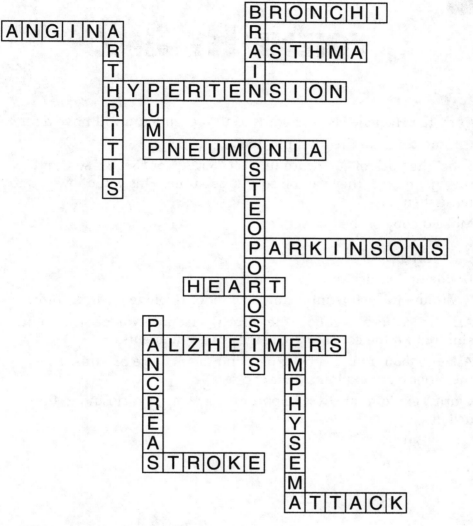

Across

1. bronchi
2. angina
4. asthma
5. hypertension
7. pneumonia
9. Parkinson's
10. heart
12. Alzheimer's
14. stroke
15. attack

Down

1. brain
3. arthritis
6. pump
8. osteoporosis
11. pancreas
13. emphysema

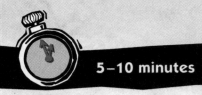

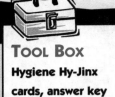

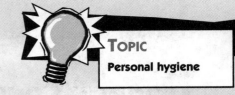

Hygiene Hy-Jinx

Preparation

1. Copy the Hygiene Hy-Jinx cards so that each team will have a set.

2. Cut the cards on the lines provided.

3. Label the back of each card in a set "Set A," or "Set B," so that if they get mixed, they will be easy to separate. This will allow you to reuse them.

4. Make a copy of the answer key.

Implementation

1. Divide the participants into two teams.

2. Distribute to each team a complete set of Hygiene Hy-Jinx cards.

3. Ask the learners to choose the correct personal hygiene statements, eliminating the cards with the incorrect statements.

4. Ask one team to begin by explaining their choice of cards. Then the other team explains their choice.

5. Clarify, explain, or stress important concepts as a closing to this activity.

EDUCATOR SECRETS:

Have group members take turns as spokesperson for their team.

By: Michele Deck, MEd, BSN, RN, ACCE-R
Nancy Hennen, BSN, RNC

HYGIENE HY-JINX

CARDS

Uniforms need to be clean.	Use name tags at all times.
No perfume.	Bathe daily.
Practice good body posture.	Uniforms need to fit well.
Limit jewelry.	Brush teeth after meals.
Moderate makeup.	Use deodorants.
Wear comfortable shoes; keep them clean and white.	Get enough sleep.
Never take alcohol or drugs before going to work.	Wear large hoop earrings.
Hair needs to be simple, clean, and off the shoulders.	Once everyone knows you, you don't need to wear a name tag.
Your patients will know you are well groomed by the odor of your cologne.	

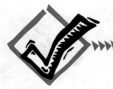

Hygiene Hy-Jinx

Answer Key

Uniforms need to be clean.	Use name tags at all times.
No perfume.	Bathe daily.
Practice good body posture.	Uniforms need to fit well.
Limit jewelry.	Brush teeth after meals.
Moderate makeup.	Use deodorants.
Wear comfortable shoes; keep them clean and white.	Get enough sleep.
Never take alcohol or drugs before going to work.	Wear large hoop earrings. INCORRECT
Hair needs to be simple, clean, and off the shoulders.	Once everyone knows you, you don't need to wear a name tag. INCORRECT
Your patients will know you are well groomed by the odor of your cologne. INCORRECT	

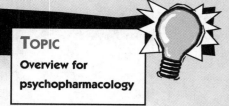

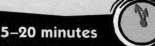
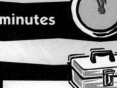

PSYCHOPHARMACOLOGY CROSSWORD PUZZLE

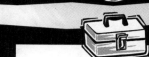

Preparation

1. Make a copy of the ready-to-use Psychopharmacology crossword puzzle for each participant.

2. Use this as an introduction to the lesson or as a review after the lesson.

3. Make sure each participant has a pen or pencil.

4. Make a copy of the answer key.

Variation

1. Use a poster printer copy machine to turn the crossword into a poster-size image.

2. Plan for groups of two to six to discuss and fill in a poster-size copy of the crossword puzzle before or after your lesson.

Implementation

1. Pass out the large or small crossword puzzle.

2. Challenge your learners to complete the puzzle as individuals or as teams.

3. If energy and attention are low during your lesson presentation, stop and let your participants engage in this energizing activity.

4. Crossword puzzles can also be sent out days or weeks after the lesson as reinforcement of important concepts.

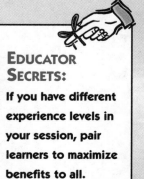

EDUCATOR
SECRETS:

If you have different
experience levels in
your session, pair
learners to maximize
benefits to all.

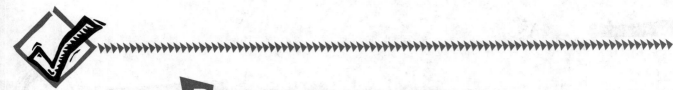

PSYCHOPHARMACOLOGY CROSSWORD PUZZLE

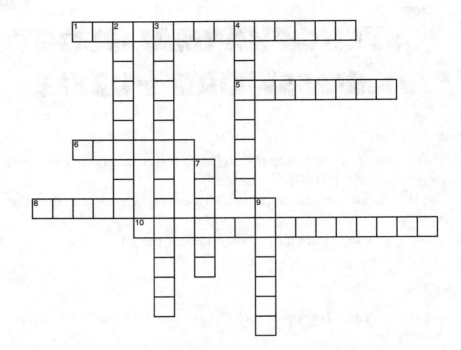

Across

1. General term for particular side effects of antipsychotics; dystonia is one

5. The amino acid that patients on 8 Across must avoid

6. Antipsychotic medication, also called major tranquilizers and neuroleptics; others in same group are Thorazine, Mellaril

8. One of three major categories of antidepressants; includes Nardil, Parmate, Marplan; must follow diet restrictions (abbrev. plural)

10. The common category of minor tranquilizers

Down

2. One of three major categories of antidepressants; includes Elavil, Ascendin, Tofranil; highly lethal in overdose

3. Type of effect seen with the tricyclics, characterized by orthostatic hypotension, blurred vision, sedation, dry mouth, etc.

4. Intense restlessness

7. One of the second generation antidepressants; the object of recent scrutiny due to possible paradoxical reactions it may cause

9. Primary medication for Bipolar Affective Disorder; interacts with patient's sodium level

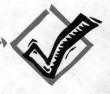

PSYCHOPHARMACOLOGY CROSSWORD PUZZLE

ANSWER KEY

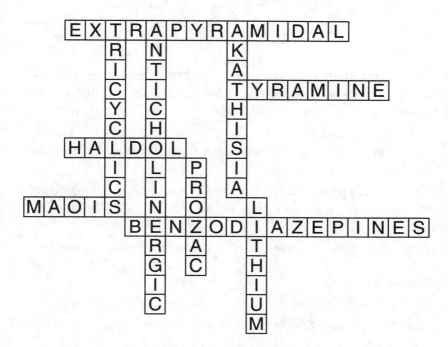

Across

1. extrapyramidal
5. tyramine
6. Haldol
8. MAOIs
10. benzodiazepines

Down

2. tricyclics
3. anticholinergic
4. akathisia
7. Prozac
9. lithium

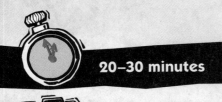

TOOL BOX

Tic Tac Toe board, *X* and *O* squares, small reward

TOPIC

Ostomy care, air mattress, low air loss bed, blue pads, foot drop, eggcrate, skin care, body aligners, positioning, diapers

TIC TAC TOE

Preparation

1. Create a game board on poster paper containing three rows of three categories each, using the ready-to-use Tic Tac Toe game board as a model. (You can also make an overhead transparency.)

2. Copy the five *X* and five *O* Tic Tac Toe playing pieces to the same size as the category square listed on the poster board (or overhead transparency).

3. Cut the playing pieces apart on the lines. If using poster board, attach tape, velcro, or an adhesive substance to the back of the *X*s and *O*s.

4. Copy the Category Questions and Answers for your reference.

Implementation

1. Divide the group into two teams, one *X* and one *O*.

2. One team begins by picking a category name.

3. The instructor asks a corresponding question.

4. If the group answers the question correctly, it puts the symbol their team selected (*X* or *O*) on that spot.

5. The opposing team then takes a turn answering a question. The first team to get three horizontally, vertically, or diagonally wins the game.

EDUCATOR SECRETS:

Play more than one game to cover all the information.

By: Michele Deck, MEd, BSN, RN, ACCE-R
Nancy Hennen, BSN, RNC

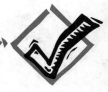

Tic Tac Toe

Game Board

Directions: This playing board can be made into an overhead transparency or poster.

Clouds	**Marshmallows**	**Blue Lagoon**
Foam Facts	**Rafting**	**Line Up**
Laid Back	**Attends-tion!!!**	**Baby Soft**

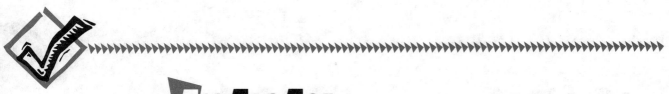

Tic Tac Toe

Game Board Playing Pieces

X	X	X
X	X	X
O	O	O
O	O	O

Tic Tac Toe

Category Questions and Answers

Rafting (Ostomy Care)

(Middle Category)

1. What is a surgical opening made in the large intestine? (*Colostomy*)

2. What is a surgical opening made in the small intestine? (*Ileostomy*)

3. What is a surgical opening made to drain urine from the body? (*Urostomy*)

1. When you clean around an ostomy, what may occur? (*Slight bleeding. Notify your nurse if it becomes excessive.*)

2. How often do you need to change a colostomy and an ileostomy pouch? (*Every three to four days*)

3. How full should a colostomy or an ileostomy pouch be when you empty them? (*One third full*)

1. What do you inspect the skin around an ostomy for? (*Breakdown, redness, or blistering*)

2. What do you always need to save when changing or emptying an ostomy pouch? (*The clamp*)

3. What do you need to hold over a urostomy stoma while you are changing the pouch and why? (*A 4 x 4 gauze wick to prevent leakage*)

continued

233

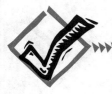

TIC TAC TOE   *continued*

CATEGORY QUESTIONS AND ANSWERS

Attends-tion!!! (Diapers)

1. How often should the diaper be checked for saturation? (*Frequently*)

2. True or false: The diaper should usually be removed when a patient is put to bed. (*True*)

3. If the diaper is left on when a patient is in bed, how should it be placed? (*Spread out flat on the bed*)

Baby Soft (Skin Care)

1. Skin needs to be kept clean and dry. What three things do you do after each episode of incontinence or in daily bathing? (*Use a mild soap, rinse well, and dry well.*)

2. When you inspect the skin, what do you look for? (*Dry, flaky areas, red or broken areas*)

3. A moisture barrier ointment is used to protect the skin from outside irritants. How much do you use? (*A thin coat. Sometimes a cornstarch powder is sprinkled on and the excess is dusted off. This will help absorb excess moisture.*)

Blue Lagoon (Blue Pads)

1. How many blue pads do you use at a time under the patient? (*Only one blue pad. You should never place multiple layers of blue pads and sheets under the patient.*)

2. At what level of the body do you place a blue pad? (*At the waist level*)

3. True or false: Blue pads are not necessary underneath the head or the feet unless drainage is present. (*True*)

Clouds (Low Air Loss Bed)

1. True or false: with the low air loss bed, the company will provide special sheets. (*True*)

2. Other than special sheets, what else does the low air loss bed company provide? (*Blue pads or low air loss bed incontinence pads*)

3. Who sets up and picks up the low air loss bed? (*The company representative*)

continued

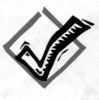

TIC TAC TOE *continued*

CATEGORY QUESTIONS AND ANSWERS

Foam Facts (Foot Drop Stop/Eggcrate)

1. What is a foam device used to elevate the foot off the mattress? (*Foot drop stop*)

2. What is a foam device used only for comfort, not relief of pressure? (*Eggcrate*)

3. What device allows you to rotate the legs inward or outward? (*Foot drop stop*)

Laid Back (Positioning)

1. If the patient is at high risk for skin breakdown, how often should he or she be turned? (*Every two hours*)

2. Should a patient be turned if he or she is on a pressure relieving device? (*Yes, every two hours*)

3. If a patient is on his or her side, how should his or her legs be positioned? (*His or her legs should be slightly bent at the knees. Place a pillow between his or her knees and a body aligner at his or her back.*)

Line Up (Body Aligners)

1. What is a foam wedge device used to maintain a patient's position in bed? (*Body aligner*)

2. What device can be used as a foot board? (*Body aligner*)

3. True or false: A body aligner should be placed in a pillowcase before patient use. (*False*)

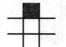

Marshmallows (Air Mattress)

1. What section of the air mattress can be removed and be placed in a chair for the patient to sit on? (*Foot section*)

2. True or false: An air mattress is disposable. (*False. Place it in a bag and place it in the dirty utility room.*)

3. When you make a bed with an air mattress, where do you tuck the bottom and draw sheets? (*Under the air mattress*)

235

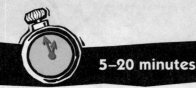

5–20 minutes

TOOL BOX

Substance Misuse
and Abuse crossword
puzzle, pens or
pencils, answer key

SUBSTANCE MISUSE AND ABUSE CROSSWORD PUZZLE

Preparation

1. Make a copy of the ready-to-use Substance Misuse and Abuse crossword puzzle for each participant.

2. Use this as introduction to the lesson or as a review after the lesson.

3. Make sure all participants have a pen or pencil.

4. Make a copy of the answer key.

Variation

1. Use a poster printer copy machine to turn the crossword into a poster-size image.

2. Plan for groups of two to six to discuss and fill in a poster-size copy of the crossword puzzle before or after your lesson.

Implementation

1. Pass out the large or small crossword puzzle.

2. Challenge your learners to complete the puzzle as individuals or as teams.

3. If energy and attention are low during your lesson presentation, stop and let your participants engage in this energizing activity.

4. Crossword puzzles can also be sent out days or weeks after the lesson as reinforcement of important concepts.

EDUCATOR SECRETS:

If you have different
ability levels in your
session, pair learners
to maximize benefits
to all.

From Instructor's Resource Manual/Test Bank
for *Mosby's Pharmacology in Nursing*, ed 18,
St. Louis, 1992, Mosby.

Substance Misuse and Abuse Crossword Puzzle

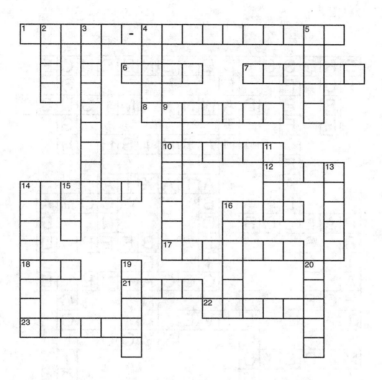

Across

1. Situation in which a drug is capable of relieving withdrawal symptoms of another drug
6. Initials for federal agency that monitors data on drug abuse
7. Indiscriminate use of drugs
8. Form of cannabis
10. Symptom of cocaine abuse
12. Often occurs when combining drugs
14. Symptom of heroin abuse
16. Alcoholic beverage often abused by teenagers
17. Related to the belladonna alkaloids
18. Phencyclidine
21. Can do this if person stops abusing
22. Frequently abused OTC drug
23. Pinpoint pupil

Down

2. Street name for nitrite inhalants
3. Combination of heroin and cocaine
4. Severe toxicity can lead to this
5. Symptom of ethanol abuse
9. Often abused by young athletes
11. Occurs with increases of steroids
13. Drug use leading to dependence
14. Continuing erections
15. A hallucinogenic drug
16. An alcoholic beverage
19. Symptom of amphetamine abuse
20. Symptom of morphine abuse

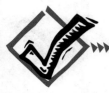

SUBSTANCE MISUSE AND ABUSE CROSSWORD PUZZLE

ANSWER KEY

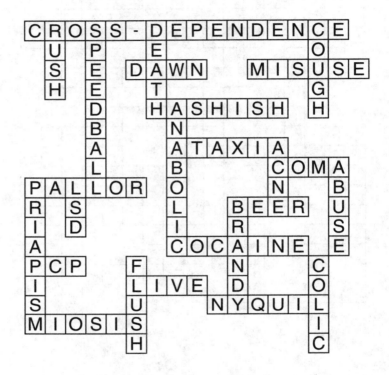

Across

1. cross-dependence
6. DAWN
7. misuse
8. hashish
10. ataxia
12. coma
14. pallor
16. beer
17. cocaine
18. PCP
21. live
22. Nyquil
23. miosis

Down

2. rush
3. speedball
4. death
5. cough
9. anabolic
11. acne
13. abuse
14. priapism
15. LSD
16. brandy
19. flush
20. colic

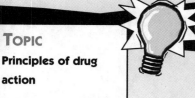

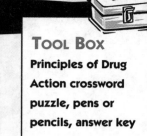

PRINCIPLES OF DRUG ACTION CROSSWORD PUZZLE

Preparation

1. Make a copy of the ready-to-use Principles of Drug Action crossword puzzle for each participant.
2. Use this as introduction to the lesson or as a review after the lesson.
3. Make sure all participants have a pen or pencil.
4. Make a copy of the answer key.

Variation

1. Use a poster printer copy machine to turn the crossword puzzle into a poster-size image.
2. Plan for groups of two to six to discuss and fill in a poster-size copy of the crossword puzzle before or after your lesson.

Implementation

1. Pass out the large or small crossword puzzle.
2. Challenge your learners to complete the puzzle as individuals or as teams.
3. If energy and attention are low during your lesson presentation, stop and let your participants engage in this energizing activity.
4. Crossword puzzles can also be sent out days or weeks after the lesson as reinforcement of important concepts.

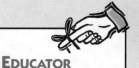

EDUCATOR SECRETS:
If you have different ability levels in your session, pair learners to maximize benefits to all.

From Instructor's Resource Manual/Test Bank for *Mosby's Pharmacology in Nursing*, ed 18, St. Louis, 1992, Mosby.

PRINCIPLES OF DRUG ACTION
CROSSWORD PUZZLE

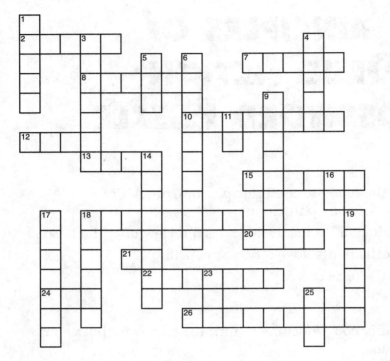

Across

2. A way to administer medications
7. Organic substance insoluble in water
8. Liquid part of the blood
10. Objective or subjective effect of a drug
12. A factor affecting the dose of medications for a child
13. Area in which inhalants are absorbed
15. Environment that increases the absorption of aspirin
18. Movement of a drug in the body is called pharmaco-_____
20. The fundamental unit of all living organisms
21. The initials for *therapeutic index*
22. A form in which a drug can be taken orally
24. A factor affecting the effects of a drug
26. Term for the process of ridding the body of a drug

Down

1. Another term for medications
3. A route in which medications are applied to the skin
4. Various places where drugs can be injected
5. Abbrev. Aspirin (abbrev.)
6. Adverse reaction produced unintentionally
9. The smallest amount of a substance that can exist alone
11. Initials for a route in which a drug is instilled in tissue
14. Factors we are born with that can affect drug effects
16. The initials for a route in which a drug is instilled in muscle
17. An organ that aids in absorption of a drug
18. An organ that can eliminate drugs
19. Pharmacodynamics of a drug
23. A factor affecting the metabolism of a drug
25. A form in which a drug can be applied to the skin

Principles of Drug Action Crossword Puzzle

Answer Key

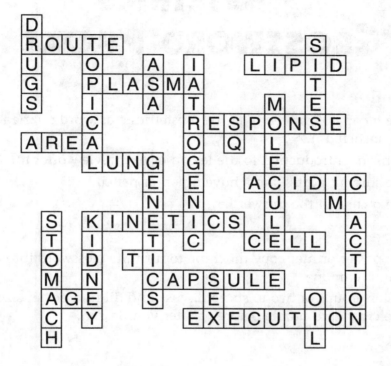

Across

2. route
7. lipid
8. plasma
10. response
12. area
13. lung
15. acidic
18. kinetics
20. cell
21. TI
22. capsule
24. age
26. excretion

Down

1. drugs
3. topical
4. sites
5. ASA
6. iatrogenic
9. molecule
11. SQ
14. genetics
16. IM
17. stomach
18. kidney
19. action
23. sex
25. oil

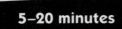
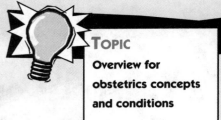
OBSTETRICS CROSSWORD PUZZLE

Preparation

1. Make a copy of the ready-to-use Obstetrics crossword puzzle for each participant.
2. Use this as introduction to the lesson or as a review after the lesson.
3. Make sure all participants have a pen or pencil.
4. Make a copy of the answer key.

Variation

1. Use a poster printer copy machine to turn the crossword into a poster-size image.
2. Plan for groups of two to six to discuss and fill in a poster-size copy of the crossword puzzle before or after your lesson.

Implementation

1. Pass out the large or small crossword puzzle.
2. Challenge your learners to complete the puzzle as individuals or as teams.
3. If energy and attention are low during your lesson presentation, stop and let your participants engage in this energizing activity.
4. Crossword puzzles can also be sent out days or weeks after the lesson as reinforcement of important concepts.

EDUCATOR SECRETS:
If you have different ability levels in your session, pair learners to maximize benefits to all.

OBSTETRICS CROSSWORD PUZZLE

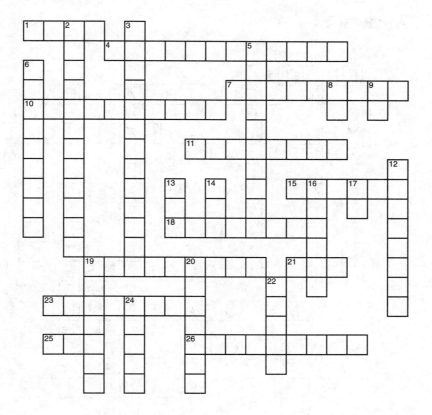

Across

1. _____ metrium; inner lining of uterus
4. Cyclic vaginal discharge; occurs from puberty to menopause
7. Prolapse or herniation of the rectum
10. Contraceptive used to immobilize or destroy sperm
11. Encapsulated connective tissue tumors
15. Upper portion of the uterus
18. Uterus and umbilical cords unfortunately do this
19. Permanent cessation of menstrual cycles
21. Intrauterine device (abbrev.)
23. Round, female type pelvis
25. Stimulates development of Graafian follicle (abbrev.)
26. Periodic reopening and discharge of ovum from the ovary

Down

2. Difficult or painful menstruation
3. Union of an ovum and a sperm
5. Absence of menstruation
6. Bladder herniation
8. Distance between upper margin, superior, border of symphysis pubis to sacral promontory (abbrev.)
9. Hormone that stimulates ovulation (abbrev.)
12. Female hormone produced by ovaries and placenta
13. Papanicolaou, as in smear (abbrev.)
14. _____ metrium, smooth muscle of the uterus
16. Muscular organ of female reproduction
17. Distance between sacral promontory and lower margin of symphysis pubis (abbrev.)
19. Bills are paid this way; also the frequency of uterine lining replacement
20. Male type pelvis
22. Score; numerical expression of infant's condition 1, 5, 15 min.
24. Produces the female reproduction cell

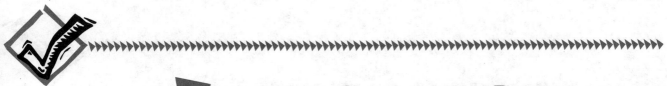

Obstetrics Crossword Puzzle

Answer Key

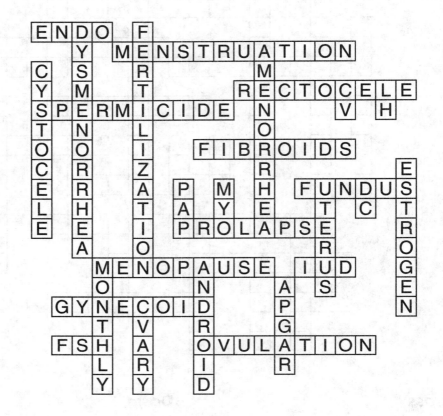

Across

1. endo
4. menstruation
7. rectocele
10. spermicide
11. fibroids
15. fundus
18. prolapse
19. menopause
21. IUD
23. gynecoid
25. FSH
26. ovulation

Down

2. dysmenorrhea
3. fertilization
5. amenorrhea
6. cystocele
8. CV
9. LH
12. estrogen
13. PAP
14. MYO
16. uterus
17. DC
19. monthly
20. android
22. Apgar
24. ovary

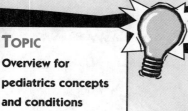
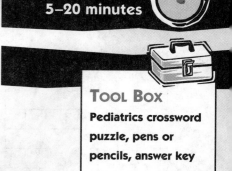

TOOL BOX
Pediatrics crossword
puzzle, pens or
pencils, answer key

PEDIATRICS CROSSWORD PUZZLE

Preparation

1. Make a copy of the ready-to-use Pediatrics crossword puzzle for each participant.
2. Use this as introduction to the lesson or as a review after the lesson.
3. Make sure all participants have a pen or pencil.
4. Make a copy of the answer key.

Variation

1. Use a poster printer copy machine to turn the crossword into a poster-size image.
2. Plan for groups of two to six to discuss and fill in a poster-size copy of the crossword puzzle before or after your lesson.

Implementation

1. Pass out the large or small crossword puzzle.
2. Challenge your learners to complete the puzzle as individuals or as teams.
3. If energy and attention are low during your lesson presentation, stop and let your participants engage in this energizing activity.
4. Crossword puzzles can also be sent out days or weeks after the lesson as reinforcement of important concepts.

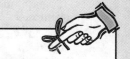

EDUCATOR SECRETS:
If you have different
ability levels in your
session, pair learners
to maximize benefits
to all.

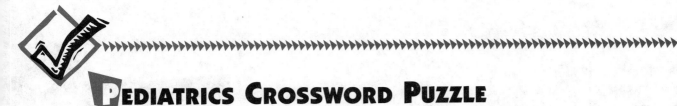

PEDIATRICS CROSSWORD PUZZLE

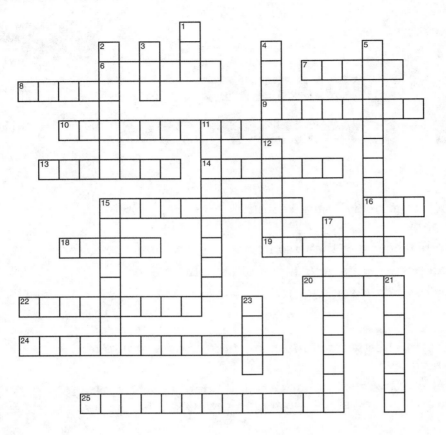

Across

6. Type of immunity stemming from antibodies and formed as a result of having a communicable disease
7. National Council Licensure Exam (abbrev.)
8. After puberty, sterility in males is the major complication of this disease
9. Major nursing intervention for prevention of STDs
10. Varicella zoster
13. Exanthema subitum
14. Disease has adverse effect on fetus during first trimester
15. Specialty concerned with health and disease in children
16. Eyes allow us to do this
18. Washing these is the most important way to reduce the spread of infection
19. Document received after successful completion of NCLEX
20. "Critters" that transmit Rocky Mountain Spotted Fever
22. Most commonly reported STD
24. Serious complication after viral infection
25. Drug of choice in febrile children during viral illness

Down

1. Human immunodeficiency virus (abbrev.)
2. Immunity type formed outside the body
3. Communicable disease transmitted by direct genital-sexual contact (abbrev.)
4. Term child uses to describe his/her skin lesion
5. Lice infestation
11. Mumps
12. Old-fashioned instrument used when taking NCLEX
15. Parasite that infects GI tract causing severe anal itching
17. Used to treat gonorrhea and syphilis
21. Type of fever caused by beta hemolytic streptococcus group A
23. Tick-borne disease characterized by flu-like symptoms

Pediatrics Crossword Puzzle

Answer Key

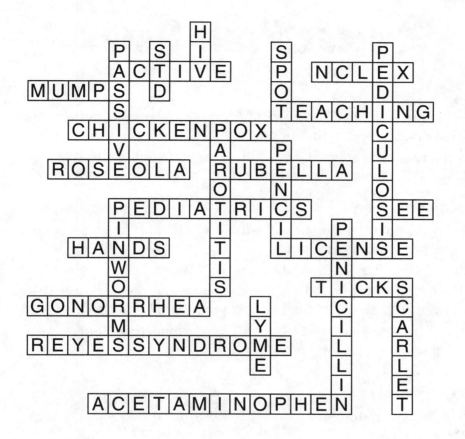

Across

6. active
7. NCLEX
8. mumps
9. teaching
10. chickenpox
13. roseola
14. rubella
15. pediatrics
16. see
18. hands
19. license
20. ticks
22. gonorrhea
24. Reyes syndrome
25. acetaminophen

Down

1. HIV
2. passive
3. STD
4. spot
5. pediculosis
11. parotitis
12. pencil
15. pinworms
17. penicillin
21. scarlet
23. Lyme

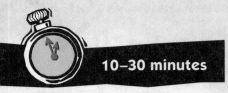

10–30 minutes

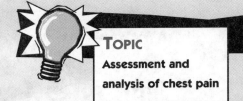
TOOL BOX
Index cards,
stethoscopes,
comfortable attire

CHEST PAIN PAIRS

Preparation

1. Write one sample disease per index card, assuring that there is at least one card per participant.

2. Copy the ready-to-use Chest Pain Pairs Differential Analysis of Chest Pain sheet so that each participant has one for reference.

Implementation

1. Following a discussion of assessing and differentiating chest pain, have participants group into pairs.

2. Distribute "disease cards" to each participant.

3. Ask half the learners to act like they have the disease while their partners assess and differentiate a probable diagnosis.

4. The partners then switch. (Make sure partners have different diagnoses.)

Sample diseases:

Psychogenic regional
   pain syndrome
Unstable angina
Pulmonary embolus
Tertz's syndrome
Angina
Myocardial infarction

Rib trauma
Aortic dissection
Esophageal pain
Overuse syndrome
Pericarditis
Asthma
Pneumonia

**EDUCATOR
SECRETS:**
Use a handout to
help learners choose
the correct disease
state.

By: Regina Lawless Phelps, MN, RN

CHEST PAIN PAIRS

DIFFERENTIAL ANALYSIS OF CHEST PAIN

Disorder	Location	Quality	Duration	Associated Phenomena	Medication
Angina	Chest with radiation	Tight, squeezing pressure, heavy	Less than 30 minutes; recurrent	Activity related palpitations, dizzy, dyspnea, weakness	NTG
MI	Anterior chest with radiation	Vise-like, crushing, choking	30 minutes and up	Nausea, vomiting, diaphoresis, syncope, palpitations, dyspnea	Morphine, narcotics IV, NTG, streptokinase
Pericarditis	Chest	Sharp, stabbing	Varies	Nonspecific	Not easily relieved
Pulmonary embolus	Chest	Sharp, pleuritic, related to respirations	Varies	Hx of vessel injury, tachy-cardia, SOB, hemoptysis, ABG alterations	Narcotic
Aortic dissection	Midline chest	Sudden, severe, tearing, ripping	Sudden, constant	New murmur, loss of adequate circulation to extremities	Surgery
GI disease	Epigastrum to upper chest	Burning, sharp	Variable, recurrent	Related to meals, activity	Antacids; antispasmodics
Chest wall	Chest	Dull, aching, locally tender	Recurrent, variable	Nonexertional	ASA, non-steroidals
Prolapsed mitral valve	Chest	Sharp, brief	Recurrent	Nonexertional, variable click-murmur systolic	None

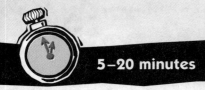

TOOL BOX
Overview of the
Blood crossword
puzzle, pens or
pencils, answer key

OVERVIEW OF THE BLOOD CROSSWORD PUZZLE

Preparation

1. Make a copy of the ready-to-use Overview of the Blood crossword puzzle for each participant.
2. Use this as introduction to the lesson or as a review after the lesson.
3. Make sure all participants have a pen or pencil.
4. Make a copy of the answer key.

Variation

1. Use a poster printer copy machine to turn the crossword into a poster-size image.
2. Plan for groups of two to six to discuss and fill in a poster-size copy of the crossword puzzle before or after your lesson.

Implementation

1. Pass out the large or small crossword puzzle.
2. Challenge your learners to complete the puzzle as individuals or as teams.
3. If energy and attention are low during your lesson presentation, stop and let your participants engage in this energizing activity.
4. Crossword puzzles can also be sent out days or weeks after the lesson as reinforcement of important concepts.

EDUCATOR SECRETS:
If you have different
ability levels in your
session, pair learners
to maximize benefits
to all.

From Instructor's Resource Manual/Test Bank
for *Mosby's Pharmacology in Nursing,* ed 18,
St. Louis, 1992, Mosby.

Overview of the Blood Crossword Puzzle

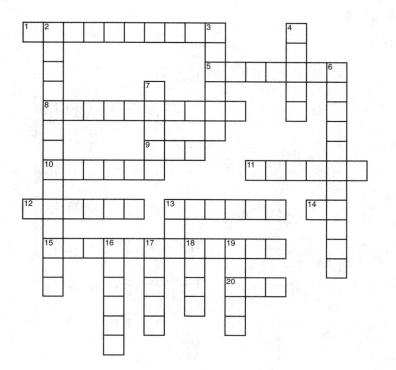

Across

1. Cell that fights infection
5. Protein that helps maintain osmolality
8. Combines with oxygen
9. Hematocrit (abbrev.)
10. Fluid portion of the blood
11. A chemical substance involved with clotting
12. Combines with platelets to reinforce clots
13. Disorder caused by decreased hemoglobin
14. Antigen present on RBC
15. Another word for platelets
20. Platelet (abbrev.)

Down

2. Hormone produced by kidney
3. Pooling of blood
4. Fluid other than blood that carries leukocytes
6. One type of WBC
7. First letter of the Greek alphabet
13. Types of blood
16. Gas carried by RBCs
17. Fluid that circulates in arteries and veins
18. Necessary to occur to prevent hemorrhage
19. Various blood classifications

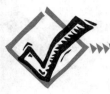

OVERVIEW OF THE BLOOD CROSSWORD PUZZLE

ANSWER KEY

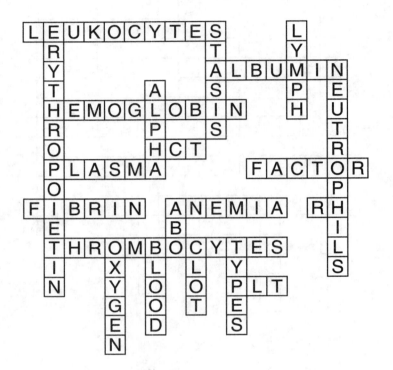

Across

1. leukocytes
5. albumin
8. hemoglobin
9. HCT
10. plasma
11. factor
12. fibrin
13. anemia
14. RH
15. thrombocytes
20. PLT

Down

2. erythropoietin
3. stasis
4. lymph
6. neutrophils
7. alpha
13. ABO
16. oxygen
17. blood
18. clot
19. types

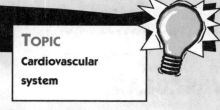
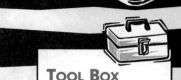
OVERVIEW OF THE CARDIOVASCULAR SYSTEM CROSSWORD PUZZLE

TOOL BOX
Overview of the
Cardiovascular
System crossword
puzzle, pens or
pencils, answer key

Preparation

1. Make a copy of the ready-to-use Overview of the Cardiovascular System crossword puzzle for each participant.
2. Use this as introduction to the lesson or as a review after the lesson.
3. Make sure all participants have a pen or pencil.
4. Make a copy of the answer key.

Variation

1. Use a poster printer copy machine to turn the crossword into a poster-size image.
2. Plan for groups of two to six to discuss and fill in a poster-size copy of the crossword puzzle before or after your lesson.

Implementation

1. Pass out the large or small crossword puzzle.
2. Challenge your learners to complete the puzzle as individuals or as teams.
3. If energy and attention are low during your lesson presentation, stop and let your participants engage in this energizing activity.
4. Crossword puzzles can also be sent out days or weeks after the lesson as reinforcement of important concepts.

EDUCATOR SECRETS:
If you have different ability levels in your session, pair learners to maximize benefits to all.

From Instructor's Resource Manual/Test Bank for *Mosby's Pharmacology in Nursing*, ed 18, St. Louis, 1992, Mosby.

OVERVIEW OF THE CARDIOVASCULAR SYSTEM CROSSWORD PUZZLE

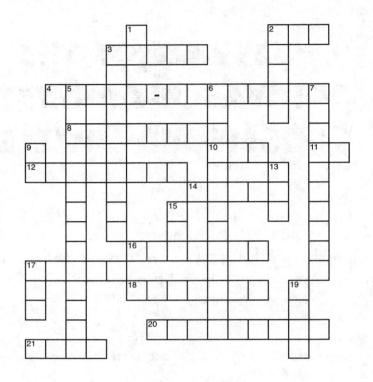

Across

2. Adenosine triphosphatase (abbrev.)
3. Major parasympathetic nerve innervation of the heart
4. Name of law pertaining to force of heart contraction
8. Fibers that are part of conduction system of heart
10. Number of ventricles and atria
11. Calcium (abbrev.)
12. Term for speed
14. Term for when heart conduction does not occur
16. Term for the period of heart contraction
17. Organ that pumps blood
18. Main cation affecting electrical stimulation of the heart
20. Stimulus that changes the resting membrane
21. Calcium, potassium, and sodium are examples

Down

1. Sodium (abbrev.)
2. Top chambers of the heart
3. Chambers that force blood to various parts of the body
5. Term for cardiac contraction recovery
6. Neurotransmitter that stimulates the vagus nerve
7. Digitalis is an example of this classification
9. Node that stimulates the heart to contract
13. Electrocardiogram; old-fashioned (abbrev.)
15. Letters on graph depicting ventricular contraction
17. Part of conduction system of the heart
19. Condition that slows down blood flow

Overview of the Cardiovascular System Crossword Puzzle

Answer Key

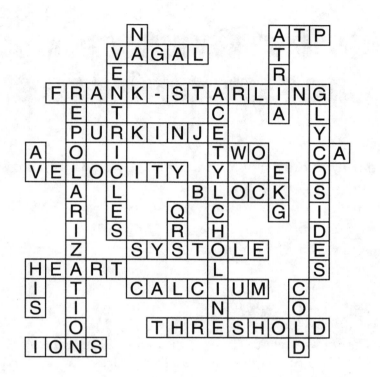

Across

2. ATP
3. vagal
4. Frank-Starling
8. Purkinje
10. two
11. CA
12. velocity
14. block
16. systole
17. heart
18. calcium
20. threshold
21. ions

Down

1. NA
2. atria
3. ventricles
5. repolarization
6. acetylcholine
7. glycosides
9. AV
13. EKG
15. QRS
17. HIS
19. cold

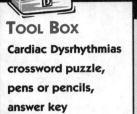

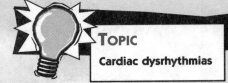

TOOL BOX

Cardiac Dysrhythmias
crossword puzzle,
pens or pencils,
answer key

CARDIAC DYSRHYTHMIAS CROSSWORD PUZZLE

Preparation

1. Make a copy of the ready-to-use Cardiac Dysrhythmias crossword puzzle for each participant.

2. Use this as introduction to the lesson or as a review after the lesson.

3. Make sure all participants have a pen or pencil.

4. Make a copy of the answer key.

Variation

1. Use a poster printer copy machine to turn the crossword into a poster-size image.

2. Plan for groups of two to six to discuss and fill in a poster-size copy of the crossword puzzle before or after your lesson.

Implementation

1. Pass out the large or small crossword puzzle.

2. Challenge your learners to complete the puzzle as individuals or as teams.

3. If energy and attention are low during your lesson presentation, stop and let your participants engage in this energizing activity.

4. Crossword puzzles can also be sent out days or weeks after the lesson as reinforcement of important concepts.

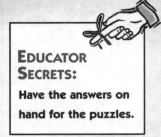

EDUCATOR SECRETS:

Have the answers on hand for the puzzles.

From Atwood S, Stanton C, and Storey J:
Introduction to Basic Cardiac Dysrhythmias,
St. Louis, 1990, Mosby.

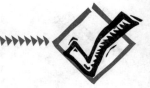

CARDIAC DYSRHYTHMIAS CROSSWORD PUZZLE

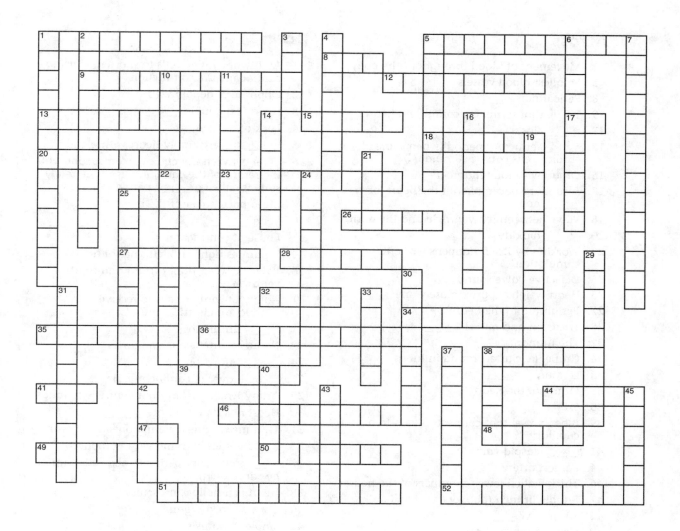

continued

CARDIAC DYSRHYTHMIAS CROSSWORD PUZZLE *continued*

Across

1. Movement of blood throughout the body
5. Smallest blood vessels
8. Pericardial _____
9. Tissue that forms sac containing heart
12. _____ fibers
13. _____ refractory period (when some cardiac cells can be stimulated)
15. Organ with four chambers
17. Secondary pacemaker of the heart, or _____ node
18. Valve between left ventricle and the aorta
20. _____ dioxide
23. Working by itself; happens without stimulation
25. Defective valve sound
26. Heart weighs approximately one _____
27. Pertaining to the heart
28. Tricuspid and mitral _____
32. The human _____
34. Grapelike clusters found in lungs
35. Carbon _____
36. Lining of the heart
38. O₂
39. Blood vessel that connects a vein to a capillary
41. _____ cuspid valve
44. Largest artery
46. Thick-walled lower chambers of the heart
47. Bundle branch (abbrev.)
48. SA and AV _____
49. Heart is make of cardiac _____
50. Breastbone
51. Ability of cardiac cells to respond to an electric stimulus
52. _____ impulse

Down

1. Ability of cardiac cells to shorten, causing cardiac muscle contraction
2. Opposite of depolarized
3. Heart is a double _____
4. Lack of oxygen
5. _____ vessels supply heart with blood
6. Time between the end of a contraction and the return of the cardiac cells to the ready state is called a _____ period
7. Main pacemaker of the heart
10. Vena _____
11. Phase of contraction
14. Separates right and left sides of heart
16. Valve between right atrium and right ventricle
19. Ability of cardiac cells to receive and conduct an electrical impulse
21. _____ atrial block
22. Connects arteries to capillaries
24. _____ infarction
25. Second layer of cardiac muscle
29. Artery leading from right ventricle to lungs
30. Heart has four separate _____
31. Thin membrane covering outside of heart
33. Blood vessels carrying waste products
37. _____ refractory period (when cells cannot be stimulated)
38. Heart is a hollow, muscular _____
40. Cone-shaped organs
42. Single Purkinje's _____
43. Valve between left atrium and left ventricle
45. Pertaining to the atrium

CARDIAC DYSRHYTHMIAS CROSSWORD PUZZLE

ANSWER KEY

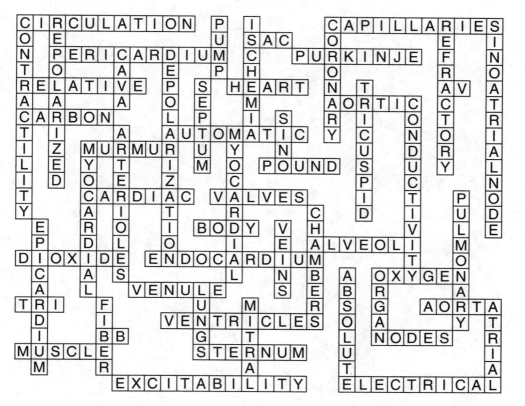

Across

1. circulation
5. capillaries
8. sac
9. pericardium
12. Purkinje
13. relative
15. heart
17. AV
18. aortic
20. carbon
23. automatic
25. murmur
26. pound
27. cardiac
28. valves
32. body
34. alveoli
35. dioxide
36. endocardium
38. oxygen
39. venule
41. tri
44. aorta
46. ventricles
47. BB
48. nodes
49. muscle
50. sternum
51. excitability
52. electrical

Down

1. contractility
2. repolarized
3. pump
4. ischemia
5. coronary
6. refractory
7. sinoatrial node
10. cava
11. depolarization
14. septum
16. tricuspid
19. conductivity
21. sino
22. arterioles
24. myocardial
25. myocardial
29. pulmonary
30. chambers
31. epicardium
33. veins
37. absolute
38. organ
40. lungs
42. fiber
43. mitral
45. atrial

PART 5

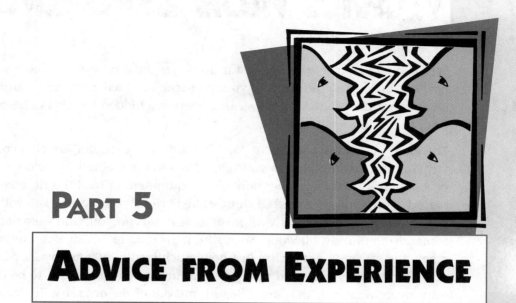

ADVICE FROM EXPERIENCE

Advice from Experience

What can you expect when you start to utilize these new tools? There will be new and surprising results from your learners. Most learners will be supportive and positive. You will discover that there are hidden benefits to be gained from using different ideas.

The ideas in this book will help you, a health care educator, develop creativity. You may be thinking to yourself, "But, I'm not creative!" The opposite is probably true. Have you ever had to use equipment or facilities that were not perfect? Have you ever worked short staffed? Have you ever worked with physicians who made nearly impossible demands on you, and were you able somehow to make it all work? Such situations require massive amounts of creativity. You may not realize just how much creativity you have used in the past. Creativity is a learned skill, not a natural talent. You learn to be creative by doing things that are different and out of the ordinary. To develop creativity, look for alternate answers to situations you face. Everyone can further develop his or her creative skills.

These tools will lead you to explore new ideas, and you might just be the person with an innovation that drastically changes how we view learning or patient teaching or curriculum in health care. Your ideas will take root and develop into a mighty force for positive change.

One measurable benefit that you will receive when you use a creative tool is better scores on evaluations at the end of your sessions. One educator I met said the best evaluation scores he ever got from learners are now his worst scores since implementing creative tools in his classes. What benefit does that give us? We will feel better about our skills as educators and increase our confidence level. Our supervisors and colleagues may see us in a different light.

Good news travels swiftly. As you have satisfied and happy educational customers, they will recommend that others attend your classes. Participants will leave a session and tell their peers that it is a must-see offering. What better way is there to directly market your value than by word of mouth? Some learners find their peers' opinions much more important than anything their boss thinks.

What benefits will you provide your learners? These tools will offer you a chance to give them personal recognition in a variety of ways. Every person responds to positive attention in an individual and unique way. Some of these tools suggest small rewards for participation; others suggest verbal recognition. Humans crave recognition for their individuality and contributions, especially in a learning situation. These tools offer opportunities to increase our learners' sense of self-esteem and accomplishment.

These activities help to break down personal and professional barriers between learners in the classroom and, then after class, back on the job. Whatever their cultural background or position, your learners will get to know their fellow learners in new ways because of these creative tools. Getting to know one another in personal ways helps to build cooperation and teamwork. Engaging in sporting and low competitive activities can create the best bonds among learners. A "we're-in-this-together" attitude can foster sharing of ideas and follow-up support after the educational session is over. Shared fun builds pleasant memories that can serve well in critical times and in the future.

What can we do to ensure success when trying these new tools? If you have only lectured in the past, you might want at first to choose one idea that sounds simple. Practice the tool with a small group of colleagues, friends, or family before you use it in a teaching setting. This gives you the opportunity to adjust and adapt the idea to your own style. Then, you can anticipate learner reactions and be ready to adapt to any situation. After using the first tool, you can then choose another and not feel the need to practice it ahead of time. Keep your explanation to the class brief, and begin with a positive attitude as if you have used this tool hundreds of times before.

What do you do in the middle of a presentation if the tool isn't working? Don't be afraid to shift gears and try something else! Assign the finish for a carryover or homework assignment. Appear as if you planned the first activity as a small break or change of pace. Simply say, "Now that we are alert and refreshed, let's continue with learning!" Some people worry that new ideas will be met with resistance. Evaluate throughout your sessions, and change what the group does not like or finds ineffective. Your positive attitude and sense of confidence that creative ideas will work is the best cue your learners have to expect success themselves.

What do you do if you have a resistant group of learners who say "We don't like games . . . . Don't make us do any!" Never refer to one of these ideas as a *game*. Call it an activity or a reinforcement of critical information. Make sure that the activity you are asking them to engage in is in their comfort zone and related to important content. Start with a low-risk idea, and as the group relaxes and starts participating, then try something more high risk. With reluctant learners, begin by using adult-type games to put them at ease about the subject before you use unfamiliar techniques. Make sure your learners know the purpose or can see the connection to what they are learning. Sometimes learners resist because they think we are wasting valuable time by doing something irrelevant to learning. These instant tools are based on what works with adult learning retention. They are not designed to be baby shower games.

Always use teams to foster competition. Some learners do not have the ego or the experience to compete alone against the rest of the class. An exception to this is in extremely small groups of one to three people. In larger groups, split your teams into sets of three to seven learners. Ask them to join forces to complete an activity and to elect a leader to take responsibility for completing the task and reporting back to you. Make it a fun responsibility for the leader and encourage team members to applaud and praise the leader.

One of the most important roles the educator can play is that of conductor of the learning orchestra. Equalize the competition so that it is fun for everyone. Make sure everyone gets a chance to participate, not just one group, and learners will feel comfortable with the activity. It is not fun or comfortable when one team is so far ahead of the others that there is no chance of anyone else catching up. You might engage in some activity that requires learners to compete against their own skills, times, or accuracy. In this way learners are not compared to each other, but to their own abilities and performance.

Always frame instant tools in a positive light. This means that the explanation of the activity should be concise, to the point, and upbeat. Apologizing about the activity or stating doubts before it begins sets a tone of failure and discontent. The positive energy and enthusiasm the educator demonstrates is directly related to the participants' reactions. Our attitude in engaging in any learning experience speaks clearly to our learners whether we are aware of it or not. Set a fun, high energy tone, and you will be pleasantly surprised at the outcome.

Stress the learning mode and rationales for these tools to left-brained learners. Give a brief reason why you have chosen a tool, and focus on learning. Some participants enjoy an activity but cannot see the educational tie to the content. Briefly explain the rationale. Once they see the relevance of a tool, they will use it as a memory tool linking content to the new approach.

Take a learning risk. We ask our learners to change their knowledge, attitudes, and skills in educational programs, but do we try to change? Some of us use methods that are routine and comfortable out of habit. In order to appreciate the commitment and energy it takes to implement learning, we may want to experience it first hand by trying one new method in each session we teach. This will directly increase our awareness and sensitivity to the needs of our learners.

Are you satisfied and comfortable with your level of teaching skills? If not, maybe it is time to invest in your own personal development by seeking to better your skills. Sharpen your ax and improve your versatility by using these and other tools for learning. Seek out opportunities to network with those who share the same goal. The synergy created can generate new possibilities for all involved. We share many challenges in health care today, and we can share some innovative solutions.

Teaching and learning can be so much fun! Finding a new tool refreshes your approach to the content and energizes everyone around you. Have you ever met someone who really enjoys what they do because they make it fun? They have that glow of satisfaction without obvious reason. They attract people because being around them makes others feel good about themselves.

The best part of using these ideas is the effect on your energy level. Instead of feeling totally drained from dragging people long distances through content, you feel refreshed. These tools add energy and creativity to the results you attain. You feel more positive when others tell you that you made a significant difference to them!

Good luck implementing your new ideas. Remember, health care learners are a special, giving group of people. Enjoy trying each and every idea in this book with them. What you do makes a positive difference in the world. You are terrific!

▶▶

If you have an idea that you are willing to share and would like to have included in Volume 2 of *Instant Teaching Tools for Health Care Educators*, please use the form on the following page. Feel free to copy the form and submit as many ideas as you would like!

Please send your ideas to:

Michele Deck

c/o Mosby

ATTN: Director of Product Acquisition and Development

Division of Continuing Education and Training

11830 Westline Industrial Drive

St. Louis, MO 63146

TOPIC

_____

_____

_____

Length of time

_____

_____
(Suggested Activity Title)

TOOL BOX

(Tools required to implement activity.)

_____

_____

_____

_____

_____

_____

_____

_____

Preparation:

_____

_____

_____

_____

_____

_____

_____

Implementation:

_____

_____

_____

_____

_____

_____

_____

_____

_____

_____

_____

_____

EDUCATOR SECRETS:

_____

_____

_____

_____

By: _____
(Source or author of activity)

Bibliography

Deck M, Silva J: *Getting adults motivated, enthusiastic and satisfied,* Minneapolis, 1990, Creative Training Techniques International.

Jensen DG: *The science of effective presentations,* Los Angeles, 1993, UCLA School of Medicine (graduate thesis).

Pike RW: *Creative training techniques handbook,* Minneapolis, 1989, Lakewood Books.